Help Me, I'm Depressed

Help Me, I'm Depressed

✦

How To Effectively Help Your Family Members, Friends, and Colleagues Dealing With Depression

Jody M. Ehrhardt Presented By Donny Lowy

iUniverse, Inc.
New York Lincoln Shanghai

Help Me, I'm Depressed
How To Effectively Help Your Family Members, Friends, and Colleagues Dealing With Depression

Copyright © 2005 by Donny Lowy

All rights reserved. No part of this book may be used or reproduced by any means, graphic, electronic, or mechanical, including photocopying, recording, taping or by any information storage retrieval system without the written permission of the publisher except in the case of brief quotations embodied in critical articles and reviews.

iUniverse books may be ordered through booksellers or by contacting:

iUniverse
2021 Pine Lake Road, Suite 100
Lincoln, NE 68512
www.iuniverse.com
1-800-Authors (1-800-288-4677)

ISBN: 0-595-34404-6

Printed in the United States of America

Contents

Foreword... vii
Introduction.. ix

Chapter 1   Recognizing Depression in Your Loved One........ 1
   What is Depression?... 1
   What Depression Isn't... 2
   The Signs and Symptoms of Depression.......................... 3

Chapter 2   How to Help Your Loved One Who is Depressed.... 7
   Finding and Then helping With Treatment....................... 7
   Help Your Loved One With Therapy.............................. 8
   Helping Your loved One With Medication Management............ 16

Chapter 3   What to Say (and Not to Say) to Someone Who is Depressed... 20
   Statements That Help... 20
   Statements That Hurt... 21

Chapter 4   What To Do When Your Loved One Is Depressed... 25

Chapter 5   What To Do If Your Loved One Refuses Your Help.. 32

Chapter 6   The Importance of Family and Friends to Someone Who Is Depressed................................. 34

Chapter 7   Taking Care Of Yourself (So You Can Take Care Of Them)... 36

Chapter 8   Who Is The Average Caregiver?.................. 44

CHAPTER 9	Avoiding Caregiver Burnout	46
CHAPTER 10	Thoughts and Concerns From Caregivers	50
CHAPTER 11	How Your Loved One Feels	55
	(Thoughts and Advice From Those Who Suffer From Depression)	55
CHAPTER 12	The Interview	60
CHAPTER 13	Resources	70
CHAPTER 14	Beyond Depression	73
About the Author		75

Foreword

The information in this book is only meant for educational purposes. Always seek professional advice before making any decisions or acting on any information. The information presented here is not meant to be offered as definitive or professional information or advice.

While this book was written with a high level of professionalism you should always verify all information contained here with a professional before making any decisions.

Introduction

Coping with and surviving the depression of a loved one can be devastating. Not only is the patient's life turned upside down but also so are the lives of everyone he or she interacts with. Depression changes every aspect of the lives of everyone it touches. Simple things such as showering, going to the store and having time to complete your work, all become huge events that have to be planned, worked through and sometimes even skipped. The carefree life you once knew will be no longer. And if your daily routine doesn't change, your emotions surely will. Gone will be the carefree over dinner chats, the good-natured "how was your day?" talks and the comfortable silences during normal routines. These things will not be gone forever, but you can expect them to replaced, at least sometimes, with strained conversation, worried thoughts and guilt during your loved one's harder times. Add to all that the facts that depression is a hard illness to understand, to have and to recover from, and you have a complicated problem. There are so many what-ifs and contingencies when dealing with depression that the day-to-day events and emotions associated with the illness become almost impossible to navigate and live through. That is where this book comes in. Through research, interviews and personal experience I have compiled a comprehensive look at what you can do to help a loved one who is struggling with depression. By using the information in this book you will be able to communicate in a more helpful manner with your loved one, communicate better with your loved one's medical professionals, act with more confidence in your decisions about their care and yours and banish feelings of guilt stemming from not knowing what to do to help. Armed with information to help ease the day to day frustrations of this illness, you will be better prepared to help the one you love (and yourself) throughout the road to recovery.

1

Recognizing Depression in Your Loved One

What is Depression?

Depression is a clinical disease, a very real medical condition like heart disease or diabetes, affecting one in every six Americans (according to the Journal of the American Medical Association). Depression occurs when certain chemicals in the brain, the ones that are responsible for controlling a person's mental state, are delivered incorrectly between brain cells. This imbalance causes real physical and emotional symptoms.

There are three major types of depression that could be affecting your loved one.

Major Depression. Major depression is defined as a severe depression that interferes with a person's work, study, sleep and everyday life. This type of depression disables the person suffering from it, causing them to be unable to function in their daily lives. This type of depression may only occur once but more often occurs several times over the course of a person's lifetime.

Dysthymia. This type of depression is usually long term but does not cause the disabling states that come with major depression. A person suffering from dysthymia will usually have chronic symptoms of depression but they are still able to function, albeit not well, in their daily lives.

Bipolar Disorder. This disorder involves reoccurring bouts of depression along with periods of mania and periods of relative normalcy. This disorder is also called manic-depressive disorder. With this disorder a sufferer will cycle between periods of highs and lows throughout their entire lives. Medications and therapy can be quite successful at controlling the "mood swings" associated with this disorder, but there is no cure for this disorder and the patient will most likely need to be in treatment (usually just medication therapy) for the rest of their lives.

Defining what depression is; is very easy, defining what causes it is not. Some theories center around the fact that depression is genetic. This theory is supported by the fact that sufferers of depression are extremely likely to have a relative that also suffered from this condition. Depression definitely stems from changes in the brain's structure and function, but it is unclear whether this abnormality is inherited or not.

Other theories cite personality traits as an indicator for developing depression. People with low self-esteem, a pessimistic attitude and a low tolerance for stress seem to have a greater predisposition to suffer from depression in some point in their lives. Whether this fact points to a psychological tendency or an early form of depression has not been determined as of yet.

A third theory as to the cause of depression points to environmental triggers. Physical illness such as stroke and cancer and life events such as the death of a loved one or lose of a job can put some people at a higher risk for developing depression.

Most often, the development of depression is the result of all three factors…genetics, personality traits and environmental factors.

What Depression Isn't.

Depression is not a character flaw. Although there is a general public view that depression is not a disease but a weakness, that if a person "just tried hard enough" the symptoms would go away, this is absolutely not true. Depression is not about being overly sensitive, lazy or sad. It cannot be caused by an unwillingness to try, it is not deserved, and it is not "easily" treated. Depression is not just a state of mind that a person could "snap out of" if they really wanted too. Although the description of what depression isn't may sound harsh, it is just as important as the description of what depression is…maybe even more important. Until people believe and understand that depression is real, sufferers of depression will continue to face ridicule and social ill will. Until everyone is educated on the facts of depression, until all people stop blaming it on weakness, sufferers of depression will feel the need to continue to hide their illness instead of speak out about it. And if no one is speaking out, then sufferers cannot learn from each other. By taking away the stigma of depression with education and "true stories", the illness can eventually be brought up and discussed for what it really it...a medical condition.

The Signs and Symptoms of Depression.

If you suspect that a friend or loved one is depressed, there are certain signs and symptoms that you can watch for to help determine your loved one's condition. As you read the list, keep in mind the fact that only a doctor can diagnosis depression. Use these symptoms only as a guideline to help you and your loved one recognize the need for an evaluation from a certified medical professional.

Feeling sad or empty: Depression can cause feelings of overall sadness but some sufferers experience periods of "nothingness"; periods were their brain does not register any emotion at all. Sufferers sometimes describe it as a feeling of emptiness in their lives or a big void.

Social Isolation: Is your loved one avoiding people or activities that he or she used to enjoy? Do they express a wish keep to themselves more often? Do they express a want to be alone? Many times, a person who is suffering from depression will not find joy in the things that used to make them happy. Sadness, or even a lack of feeling or emotion, can inhibit their sense of joy causing them to avoid situations that antagonize these feelings. Or, your loved one may feel "different" from everyone around them and wish to avoid these feelings as they may cause them to feel even worse about themselves and their situation.

Lack of Motivation: Is the person feeling lazy? Do they avoid doing even mundane chores? When a person is depressed they often lack the motivation needed to accomplish even simple things such as showering or finishing their work. It is not that they "don't want" to do these things, it is just that their brain doesn't allow them to feel the need to get them done. Many sufferers of depression describe this feeling as "physically being unable to make themselves find the strength to act". Feelings of inadequacy can also keep a depressed person from trying. Thoughts such as "Why should I bother?" or "Nothing good ever comes from my efforts." can discourage your loved one from starting or finishing, even enjoyable tasks.

Change in Sleeping Habits: Sometimes a person who is suffering from depression will sleep way too much, either because they are physically exhausted or because their brain is telling them that it is easier to stay in bed in order to avoid facing the day ahead. Other times, a person will sleep too little, unable to clear their mind of negative thoughts long enough to relax and fall asleep. Another sleep disruption caused by depression is early morning waking. Normal sleep cycles include periods of light sleep where a person may wake long enough to shift positions or check the clock. When a person is suffering from depression they may not be able to fall asleep again after a nocturnal waking due to having "too much on their minds".

Change in Appetite: For some people food can be used as a source of comfort. An increase in appetite could be brought on by a need to "feel better" or "feel comforted" by a familiar food or memory associated with that food. Also, many foods such as chocolate actually cause a feeling of well being when consumed due to the chemical release of certain hormones in the brain. This momentary sense of pleasure can result in a compulsion to overeat as the sufferer repeatedly searches out those feelings.

Some people, when in a state of depression, have no desire to eat. The act of making the food can be too big of a challenge. Or, feeling despondent, the person may see no need to eat. Lack of motivation can also play a role here. The sufferers may lack the will to force themselves to prepare a meal even though their body may be sending them signals of hunger or thirst.

Irritability or Anxiety: People suffering from depression are often anxious and irritable, especially when there doesn't seem to be a concrete reason to feel that way. Irritability is often brought on by negative thoughts and the general sense that life is horrible. The act of living with these negative thoughts day in and day out often brings on a general feeling of anger or irritability. Sometimes irritability, occurring more often than actual sadness, is the symptom you will notice in your loved one first.

Anxiety can be brought on by feelings of guilt such as "Why can't I snap out of this?" feelings of worthlessness such as "Why can't I be happy like everyone else?" and feelings of dread such as "What horrible thing is going to happen to me next?" Feelings such as these can cause a person to feel tense and afraid. Also, a person who is suffering from depression may have feeling of paranoia, they may feel that the world, you, their co-workers, everyone, is "out to get them". After a period of time, these feelings can occur so often that they eventually become habit. As time goes by and the person continues to feel anxious about day-to-day events, the brain becomes trained to feel these emotions on an everyday basis and the anxiety itself becomes a trigger for more anxiety.

Indecisiveness: People who are suffering from depression often experience the inability to concentrate and make decisions. Depression impairs a person's ability to think clearly, causing a "feeling of fogginess" or haziness in their thought process. As the sufferer attempts to concentrate, whether it is on work or a simple television program, their mind wanders to other, usually negative, thoughts. And their decision-making difficulty can stem from a lack of hope for the future, a belief that everything they do is doomed anyway, or the inability to concentrate on the facts long enough to make an educated decision.

Physical symptoms: Many people who suffer from depression also suffer from unexplained physical symptoms such as headaches or upset stomachs. These pains are always real but cannot be explained by a doctor or further testing. These physical pains are often brought on by the psychological symptoms involved with depression. Usually, these aches or chronic pains will lessen or disappear with proper treatment for depression.

Thoughts of death or suicide: If your loved one ever mentions having thoughts of death or he or she threatens suicide, you need to take them very seriously and seek help immediately. Talk of death or suicide can be a call for help or a way for your loved one to lessen the guilt they feel about what they are about to do. Either way, you must take any mention of death seriously. Call your loved one's doctor or take them to your local emergency room as soon as possible. Do not try to talk your loved through these thoughts yourself.

The symptoms of depression are varied and not every one suffering from depression will exhibit the same signs or even the most signs all the time. If someone you love or care about is exhibiting at least three of these signs consistently for longer than two weeks then you should talk to them about getting help. Depression is a very treatable disease and no one should have to live with the symptoms.

Once you have decided that your loved one may be depressed, it may be just as complicating to get them to seek help. In most cases, the depression itself will keep a person from seeking help. The thought of searching out help can be overwhelming. Or, a person could believe that there is no help for the way they are feeling. In these cases it could be up to you to search out a respected, qualified doctor and make the appointment for them.

2

How to Help Your Loved One Who is Depressed

Finding and Then helping With Treatment

First, know that depression can be treated. Studies show that more than eighty percent of people suffering from depression can be successfully treated. And better yet, that treatment does not have to be long-term or expensive. The most common treatment for depression includes the use of an anti-depressant medication and short-term, one-on-one counseling usually consisting of only ten to twenty visits.

To find the recommended treatment, most people who are faced with depression or the depression of a loved one start with a general check-up with their family physician. This is a great place to start for two reasons.

One, sometimes the symptoms of depression can mask or mimic the symptoms of another medical condition. It is best to schedule an appointment with a doctor to rule out any other physical causes or conditions. This visit should include a general physical exam, a complete medical history and lab tests.

Two, your general practitioner or family doctor can recommend further testing or treatment from a therapist or psychologist if the tests rule out any other physical problems or illnesses. This can be especially helpful for insurance purposes. Many insurance companies require a referral before a patient is allowed to seek mental health care.

Help Your Loved One With Therapy

In order for a person to get the full benefits of therapy they need to attend all scheduled appointments, ask questions and report all changes in behavior and thought to their doctor. This can be an overwhelming task for someone who is depressed. You can help by taking on some of these responsibilities.

First, help your loved one find a qualified doctor. Even if the family physician recommended a therapist or psychologist, that person may not "fit" with your loved one's personality or comfort level. Finding a doctor that your loved one can relate to and feel comfortable with is the first major step in assuring that they get help. Therapy only works if the patient can trust their healthcare provider enough to open up to them honestly about their feelings and trust in them enough to follow their instructions. In order to assure a good doctor/patient relationship you will need to research and interview a few doctors first.

Start with a list of recommended doctors and have your loved one narrow the list based on their general preferences. If your loved one can't help or doesn't want to help with this step then use your knowledge of the patient's preferences to narrow done the list. Would your loved one be more comfortable with a male or female doctor? Would he or she feel more comfortable with a younger doctor or an older, maybe more experienced, one? Some people feel better talking to a doctor that is close to their own age or older. Older people especially can be intimidated by the thought of trusting a younger doctor. Also, many patients find it easier to open up to a person they see as a peer.

Next, narrow done the list with general criteria. How far are you or your loved one willing to drive to see a doctor? If the trip is time consuming or out of the way, the patient may use that as an excuse not to go. Or, if you will be doing the driving, you may find that time constraints prevent you from traveling too far. How available is the doctor? Does he have evening appointments? An after hours phone number? Availability on weekends or for emergencies? In the first weeks or even months of treatment, you or your loved one may need to see him or call him more frequently. Finding an office with flexible hours makes seeking treatment easier, and easier treatment helps ensure longevity in treatment. Does the doctor have experience helping patients similar in age, background or diagnosis to your loved one? Obviously a doctor experienced with teen depression would not be of as much help to your 43-year-old spouse. Also, a doctor with similar patient backgrounds will have more knowledge about your loved one's personal feelings as he will have heard similar descriptions before.

After you have narrowed the list down to two or three doctors, call and make an appointment to meet with each of them for an informal interview. It is best if your loved one is involved with this process but if they are having doubts or dragging their feet, then you may have to go alone to this appointment. Explain on the phone your intentions and specifically state what your expectations from the meeting will be. Explain that you are interviewing doctors to treat your loved one's depression and inform them if your loved one will not be present at the meeting. Sometimes, instead of a face-to-face visit, the doctor will prefer to interview over the phone. Of course, in person visits are best, but a phone interview can also help.

Before the visit write down your questions and concerns. This will ensure that all of your questions are addressed and will cut down on the actual meeting time as you will not have to search you mind for additional questions or missed concerns. You do not want to feel rushed during this interview but you do need to be mindful of the doctor's time, especially since you may choose not to see him/her again. By using common sense and the following sample questions, you should be able to determine a "good fit" within a standard 45-minute appointment.

How long have you been in practice? This is important for obvious reasons, the longer a doctor has been in practice, the more knowledge you would have expected him to acquire. But keep in mind that the opposite can also be true. If a doctor is newer to the practice of mental health, his schooling is fresher in his mind and he may have been taught more up-to-date information in his recent studies. You might also inquire as to how much continuing education the doctor has received in the area of depression. Research and clinical studies are constantly bringing to light new information and better treatment options for depression. If your doctor keeps abreast of this new information, he will be better equipped to help your loved one.

What types of patients do you currently see? Use this question to determine the doctor's patient experience. Again, finding a doctor with patients similar to your loved one can make treatment easier and faster.

Will the patient always see you or do you rotate with another physician? This question is especially important because sometimes in bigger practices or teaching hospitals, a doctor may rotate patients with another doctor or your loved one may just see whoever is available at his appointment time. You want to try and avoid this scenario whenever possible. Therapy usually works best if a patient is allowed to develop a relationship and trust with his or her doctor and bouncing around from one doctor to the next can hamper or inhibit this process. Plus, you do not want to waste the first fifteen minutes of every appointment bringing the "new" doctor up to speed on your loved one's condition and progress.

What is your view on depression? Surprisingly, this is a very important question. Although you would assume that every mental health care professional would have the same view on depression, this is simply not true. Some doctor's even go as far as to treat it as a minor condition. Make sure that the doctor you choose shares your feelings about this condition, takes this condition seriously, and has a view on depression that you can respect and understand. If you start out the therapy at odds with your doctor on the causes or treatments of depression, your loved one's recovery will definitely be slowed or even halted.

What types of therapy do you start with or recommend? This question is important because it can prepare you for what is to come. Some treatments require more visits, some treatments require follow-up by the patient at home and some treatments require medications. It is helpful to know up front what might be expected of you and the patient throughout treatment. This knowledge will also help you determine whether your loved one will be willing to complete the treatment as prescribed. It would be harmful to your loved one to begin treatment, only to find out three weeks later that they are unwilling to follow the doctor's instructions. This scenario can make seeking future help extremely difficult because your loved one may become distrustful of doctors or treatment and refuse to try again.

How important do you feel medications are to a patient's recovery? This is an important question even if you have no qualms over the use of medication to treat depression. You will want a doctor that will use medication only when necessary, use as few medications as possible and one that holds the belief that the medication may not be a life-long necessity.

How much importance do you place on continuing therapy at home? This question is important because it will help you determine the doctor's approach to treatment. No matter how wonderful the treatment is at the doctor's office, your loved one will be required to make changes at home. Therapy appointments usually occupy about 45 minutes out of each week. You and your loved one will continue to deal with the depression and its symptoms at home for the other 6 days, 23 hours and fifteen minutes. It is imperative that your doctor is willing acknowledge your need to cope with these periods and be willing to help you and your loved one master techniques that can used outside the office.

How long do you feel treatment for therapy should last? This information is important to know up front because, while you understand that treatment could take several months or even years, you do not want therapy to become a crutch for your loved one. Good therapy teaches a person how to deal with their feelings and conditions and gives them the tools necessary to negotiate independently through life. Therapy should never teach them to become dependent on therapy. A good therapist knows when it is time to set a patient free.

How do you feel about seeing the patient's relatives during scheduled appointments or receiving phone calls from them between visits? This question is important because you want to feel welcomed by your loved one's doctor as you may be making and attending most of the appointments along with him or her. Also, you want to feel comfortable contacting the doctor if your loved one's condition worsens or if you just have a question or concern that can not wait until the next scheduled appointment. A good therapist will understand that treating and recovering from depression is a family affair, and will want to help the entire family heal, not just your loved one.

The information you glean during the interview from the sample questions will be extremely important, but the way that the doctor answers them can be even more important. As you ask questions make mental notes of the feelings you get from the doctor. Does he make you feel comfortable? Is he patient or hurried? Does he explain (and re-explain) his answers patiently, making sure you understand? Does he treat you as an equal or talk down to you? Do you feel as though you could trust him? Does he sound knowledgeable about your loved one's condition? Do his answers seem genuine or do they seem mechanical or rehearsed? A doctor with compassion and a true need to help your loved one can actually be far more helpful than an overly qualified doctor with no personal concern.

Once you and your loved one have interviewed a few doctors, discussed your findings and feelings and come to a decision, it is time to schedule the first therapy appointment. Once the appointment is set up, it is up to your loved one to decide if they want you to attend the first visit with them or not. If they express a need to have you there, remember that you are there for moral support only, you are not to discuss your own concerns or emotions. Wait to voice your concerns after the visit or through a phone call to the doctor at a later date. Never interrupt your loved one; even if you disagree with what they are saying or feel you need to clarify their thoughts. This is their time to share and vent, not yours. A qualified and experience doctor will be able to discern between fact and fiction in your loved one's answers. Letting your loved one answer however they may want to will better able the doctor to make a diagnosis based on your loved one's true feelings and not on your interpretation of them.

If your loved one does not want you along on their first or subsequent visits, do not take it personally or push them to change their mind. Maybe they will be more comfortable talking about their personal feelings alone, or maybe they are embarrassed to be having the feelings in the first place. Your loved one may also wish to discuss their relationship with you, or concerns they are having about your relationship due to the illness. These discussions are usually easier if your loved one is alone with the doctor or therapist.

If your loved one does choose to go alone, offer to drive them to the appointment and wait outside or run errands until the hour is up. Sometimes just knowing that someone is waiting for them can act as a big push toward finding the motivation to go through with the appointment.

Once your loved one has survived the first visit and they are agreeable to continuing the treatment, there are many things that you can do to help them stay motivated to see the treatment through. Between doctor visits, medication management and at-home therapies, the continuation and maintenance of care could become overwhelming for the patient as the weeks progress. To help lighten their load and assure compliance, try to become as involved as possible in their treatment without shadowing their every move or making them feel pressured.

Schedule appointments: Sometimes, a lack of motivation or feeling of hopelessness can keep a patient from scheduling or even keeping their doctor appointments. Offering to handle the scheduling for them takes away this burden and also aids in tracking the appointments if the patient is seeing multiple doctors. Simply ask your loved one if this would be a responsibility that they would like you to handle for them.

Attend appointments: If your loved one is comfortable with your presence at a few of his appointments, use that time to convey any changes you have noticed or questions you may have to the doctor. Just make sure that you clear the discussion with your loved one first. Sometimes patients suffering from depression will have a low trust threshold and surprising them at the visit with a discussion of their behavior could cause them to stop opening up in their talks with you, or confiding in you altogether. To avoid this, always discuss your concerns with the patient prior to the appointment and agree with and stick to any limits on topics they may set.

If your loved one doesn't want you to discuss them or their behavior with the doctor, you could always agree to attend the appointment only to help your loved one ensure that their questions are answered. Therapy sessions can be stressful for the patient causing them to forget concerns or changes that they had hoped to discuss. Make it your job to broach these topics with the doctor in order to get the conversation started. Even if you will not be present at the appointment, you can still help with this problem by discussing these concerns with your loved prior to the appointment and then making them a list of questions to take to their appointment.

Seek family therapy: Whether or not your loved one allows you to attend some therapy sessions with him, it is a great idea to seek therapy for yourself. Usually the best form of therapy for dealing with the depression of a loved one is family therapy. In this type of therapy the family, as a whole, attends each session. The focus of this therapy is to teach each family member ways to cope with the fallout of living with someone suffering from depression. In this therapy, each family member is allowed to express their concerns, emotions and areas of difficulty without fear of judgment or negative consequences. The therapist then intervenes if feelings are hurt, anger is roused or questions are asked. The therapist also takes into account the unique situations faced by each family member in order to provide concrete actions and changes the person can take to cope with the illness more productively.

Other therapies taught during family sessions include relaxation techniques, crisis management techniques for when your loved one is extremely ill and positive expression techniques to use when conversing about the depression or the adverse effects it has on the family. Family therapy is especially important to any depression treatment because the condition does not just effect the person who is suffering from it but every family member and all the areas of their lives as well.

Exercise with your loved one. Exercise is a great way for your loved one to raise their energy levels and overall feelings of well being. Exercise is proven to reduce stress, increase endorphins (feel-good chemicals) in the brain, and improve body image and feelings of self-worth.

Unfortunately, depression can make it almost impossible for a person to start or stick with any exercise program or activity. By exercising with your loved one, or in front of him in the hope that he joins in, you might be able to provide the added motivation they need to get going. Do not be disappointed though if this doesn't work. Remember that depression can cause the physical inability to accomplish things. If this is the case with your loved one, do not berate them for not trying and do not take the failure personally.

If you can entice your loved one to exercise, remember that exercise does not have to come in the form of rigid rules and routines. Gardening, walking and even shopping can require movement and provide the boost in activity they desperately need. Plus, these activities are usually easier for your loved one to handle for the very reason that they don't feel like exercise.

Help keep their daily lives on a regular schedule. People who suffer from depression often benefit from a tight routine in their daily schedules. Change and uncertainty of what will come next often cause undo worries and anxiety for those who suffer from this condition. To avoid adding undo stress to your loved one's life, try to make and adhere to a regular schedule. Attempt to wake, go to bed, eat and do errands at the same times everyday. If a change is routine will be necessary, attempt to forewarn your loved one hours or even days in advance. This advance notice will give your loved one time to deal with the emotions of change and time to neutralize any negative thoughts or concerns associated with that change.

Help your loved one negotiate for fewer work hours. Sometimes, a person's career can put undo stress on them, especially during times of high emotion or severe stress. Work with your loved one, and if necessary their employer, to negotiate a shorter work week or lighter work load. When a person is depressed they often find it hard to complete tasks or stay focused. Falling behind at work due to these symptoms can increase your loved one's stress and cause them to develop further feelings of failure and lowered self-esteem. To aid your loved one and their employer in accepting this change, stress to them that this is not a long-term arrangement, but rather a short-term fix that will become unnecessary once your loved one is feeling better.

Help your loved one reduce their overall stress levels. Whether the stress your loved one is experiencing is self-inflicted or environmental, there are concrete changes they can make to lower their feelings of stress. For environmental stress triggers such as family obligations, workloads, chore responsibilities and financial requirements, the answer could be as simple as cutting back on obligations or eliminating unnecessary activities all together. During bouts of severe depression, you may find it helpful to realize that it is not absolutely necessary to have a big family dinner every Sunday night or that the vacuuming does not necessarily have to be done twice a week. Let go of some expectations and allow yourself to let little things slide until your loved is feeling better.

Help them eliminate caffeine, sugars and alcohol from their diets. Small changes in diet can go along way toward helping your loved one fight their depression, but these changes can be hard for your loved one to make alone. Support them by offering to make the changes with them.

Caffeine and excessive sugar can have an anxiety-inducing effect on your loved one. Alcohol can diminish a medications benefits and also work against your loved one's recovery by placing them in a state of despair brought on by the mind-numbing effects of being intoxicated. Most people experience periods of sadness or anger when depressed and alcohol can exuberate these feelings. Rid the house of these items and make it a point to steer clear of social situations that involve these items until your loved one is farther along the road to recovery.

Helping Your loved One With Medication Management

Treatment for depression almost always involves the prescribing of medication. For a person who is in the midst of depression, medication management can be hard, if not impossible, to navigate. Helping with medication management can be an area where a family member's involvement is crucial.

Research recommended medication: Every medication currently on the market comes with side effects, precise dosing instructions and unique benefits. While the doctor should and will provide you and the patient with a run down of this information, it is beneficial to everyone involved to research each medication on your own. The quickest way to do this is to research each medication on the Internet at the website of its manufacturer. There you will find an easy to understand description of the medication, its dosage amounts and expected side effects.

To make your search more beneficial and easier to undertake, buy an inexpensive notebook and label it "medications" before you begin. Then use this notebook to chart the results of your search in order to make easy comparisons of multiple medications later. Include the following information for each medication:

Time needed to see any benefit. Most medications can take 4 to 6 weeks to reach an optimal level in the body, some can take up to 8 weeks or longer, therefore causing a delay in the time it takes the patient to actually feel the medication working. Knowing this information will allow you to help your loved one stick with a medication if they become convinced it isn't working.

Dosage amounts. Most medications come in an array of active ingredient strengths to ensure that each patient is getting the prescribed amount. These amounts can vary from medication to medication but common doses are 20mg, 40mg, 50mg and 100mg. Of course, the dosage could be as small as .01mg and up to 1000mg. The doctor will decide which dosage is best but you will want this information to determine two things. One, you may need to invest in a pill splitter if the medication only comes in 20mg but the doctor has prescribed 10mg for your loved one.

Two, many medications are less expensive if bought in the lowest number of pills possible. For instance, if the doctor has prescribed 30mg of a medication and the medication only comes in 10mg doses, then you would need to pay for three pills a day. Researching this information could supply you with a similar medication that will work just as well, that comes in a 30mg pill. You would then be able to take this information to the doctor and let him decide if the change could be made. Not only could this be a less expensive option, but also having less pills to take each day could increase your loved one's medication compliance.

Dosage options. Medications come in different forms such as pills, tablets, capsules and liquids. If your loved one has problems swallowing pills you will naturally want to ensure that the recommended medication comes in a liquid form or if not, that it is safe to chew or crush the tablet before digestion. With most slow release tablets, crushing or chewing the tablet is not recommended. Other medications cannot be delivered in liquid form. Knowing your options prior to accepting a medication can help your doctor make the choice that is best for your loved one.

Dosing instructions: Some medications come with specific dosing instructions such as recommendations to take the pills with meals or a full glass of water. It is important to know about and follow these dosing instructions to avoid unnecessary side effects and to ensure full benefit from the medication. Some medications require water to begin the break down of the pill, some medication can cause stomach upset if not ingested with food. Some medications cause extreme drowsiness, especially in the first few weeks of dosing, and require that the medication be taken at night or when the patient will be able to rest. Other dosing tips to look for include the need to avoid caffeine, as this can increase the actions of some medications in the body, the need to avoid alcohol, as this can offset a medication benefits or increase drowsiness, and the need to split a dose or double a dose in the beginning in order to reach a therapeutic level in the body within the timeframe prescribed. Another, relatively unknown tip involves using grapefruit juice as the liquid your loved one washes his pills down with. In clinical studies, grapefruit juice has been shown to be similar enough in make-up to certain medications to actually prevent the absorption of these medications. Ask your pharmacist if any information concerning this juice exists in the patient information for your prescribed medication.

Side effects: Write down all side effects associated with each medication. This information can be referenced frequently during the first few weeks of dosing and periodically there after to ensure that the patient's body is handling the new medication properly. Many side effects are common and expected. These side effects will usually subside after the first few weeks of dosing as your loved one's body grows accustom to the medication. But, it also helps to know the signs of major or serious side effects due to the remote chance that they may occur. If your loved one develops any signs of serious side effects, notify their doctor immediately or take them to the nearest emergency room.

*Note—a medication's side effects are studied in controlled clinical trials during the "new drug" testing period required by the FDA. Keep in mind that each side effect noted by a study volunteer during the clinical trial (even if they are the only volunteer to experience this side effect) must be documented and, later, included in the drug information sheet. This means that a volunteer could conceivably eat spicy food during the trial, experience heartburn afterward and *heartburn* would then be included as a side effect of the drug. This **does not** mean that you should not take all side effect warnings seriously, it just means that you need to keep the above information in mind when faced with three paragraphs of side effects per medication.

After research medication, you can also use this notebook to track refill dates, dates medications where prescribed and discontinued and changes in the dosage of each medication. This information can be quite helpful if you switch doctors and need to relay your loved one's medication history such as which medication have been prescribed in the past and the reasons that they were discontinued.

When filling prescriptions for your loved one always strive to fill them at the same pharmacy. This process will add an extra checkpoint that will help to ensure that two medications that could be harmful if taken together are never prescribed. Pharmacists play an active role in a patient's medication management and can answer many questions as well as dispense advice when needed.

To help keep the medications straight and ensure that they are taken as prescribed; purchase an inexpensive pill container at your local drugstore. These can be as simple as a two compartment case that houses a day and a night dosage or something more elaborate that sorts medications by the days of the week and the times of the dose. Using this type of container can also help your loved remember to take their medications on their own. The container, plus a gentle reminder from you, can go along way toward ensuring medication compliance.

3

What to Say (and Not to Say) to Someone Who is Depressed.

Statements That Help.

Conversations with someone who is suffering from depression can be strained at best, harmful or unbearable at worst. As with any situation, finding the right words can be difficult. When in doubt, keep the conversation light and remember that your role is to listen, support and offer love. Most sufferers are not going to share their feelings with you in the hopes that you can fix what troubles them. More often, they are just reaching out and searching for someone to listen and understand.

If they start the conversation and the topic is depression, strive to be compassionate and non-judgmental. Your loved one does not expect you to understand their feelings; they just want to know that they have your unconditional love and support. Listen, offer support and above all else, do not criticize.

Most times, your conversation will have nothing to do with the topic of depression. Use these times to interact as naturally as possible with your loved one. These talks can serve as a gentle reminder that you still love them and that they still interest you as a person. Familiar and even mundane daily occurrences such as a light hearted talk about a trip to the store can help sufferers of depression put their illness in perspective.

During your normal, routine chats, try to keep the conversation going. When asking questions of your loved one, ask open-ended questions so that there is less of a chance that they will withdraw from the conversation. Instead of asking "Did you have a good day?" ask something specific like

"What happened in your meeting today?" Strive to have normal, relaxed conversations with your loved one at least twice as often as conversations about their illness.

If you need to broach the subject of their illness, whether to express concerns with their progress or inquire as to how they are doing, always ask questions gently and in a non-threatening way. Even the best-intentioned questions can feel like attacks to a person who is already feeling down on themselves and guilty about not getting better. Try to start all sentences with "I" as in "I feel like this medication may not be working, how do you feel about it?" or "I've noticed that you seem more down today, is there anything I can do to help?" Phrasing the question in the correct way can take a sensitive topic, like your belief that your loved one is not working at home on his or her therapy, and turn it into a great sharing opportunity, like "I noticed you haven't had time to do your therapy. Maybe tonight we can turn off the TV and do your therapy together."

No matter what the conversation, if you act with love, offer help, avoid criticism and trust your feelings you will have no problem keeping the lines of communication open between you and your loved one.

Statements That Hurt.

This section is a little longer as there are numerous phrases of comfort often muttered from well meaning lips that in reality only work to make the life of a person suffering from depression harder. To this end, these actual phrases are listed here and are then followed by an explanation of what makes them unacceptable.

"I understand". That phrase is listed first as it is probably the most misused statement in the history of the spoken language. Bluntly put, No, you do not understand. To truly understand you would have to be depressed yourself or have to have suffered from depression in the past. Sad days and down-in-the-dumps moments do not count. The feelings brought on by isolated moments of sadness in no way compare to the life-crippling feelings of despair brought on by clinical depression. To claim you understand, when there is clearly no way that you could, can feel like a slap in the face to the sufferer. These two well meant words could cause anger or worse, feelings of isolation, because the sufferer knows that you do not understand. Instead of saying I understand, try saying things like "I am sorry", or "I wish I could do more to help", or "I hear what you are saying but I can't imagine your pain. I can not fathom how hard this must be for you to deal with". Any phrase that implies empathy and sympathy will work here instead.

"Snap out of it". Or the similar, "You could beat this if you really tried". Both statements, aside from being inconsiderate, relay the message that you do not believe that their depression is an illness. Would you tell a diabetic to "snap out of it" because you were tired of supplying and injecting their insulin? Would you tell a person who was blind that they could see if they just tried hard enough? Of course not! And for that reason it is a bad idea to say something of that nature to a person who is suffering from depression. The road to recovery from depression is hard and bumpy. It takes great effort and time. Obviously, if the answer were easy, the person wouldn't be depressed in the first place. Try to convey your belief that they need to help themselves in order to get better, with a phrase that solidifies your belief that their depression is a medical ailment.

Always remember that depressed people are not lazy, to them it is objectively obvious that their future prospects are bleak. The part of their brain that could "snap out of" a blue period is not working correctly. Sometimes, with medication, this brain activity can work again, but until then, your loved one needs understanding, not impossible directions.

"I was sad once so I…bought a new outfit, took up water aerobics, got my hair cut" and so on. This phrase doesn't work for the same simple reason stated above. Your sadness was a phase, theirs is a medical illness. While a new experience or item may give you an instant "pick-me-up" that allows you to refocus your mind and put the depressing incident behind you, a momentary fix is not going to help your loved one "cure" a medical condition. Instead of telling them what they can do to fix their depression, ask them to tell you what you can do to help.

"You have so much to be thankful for." People who are suffering from depression already know that they have a lot to be thankful for. This knowledge is part of what makes the depression so hard to deal with. They know, logically, that they have a lot of good things in their lives, but emotionally they cannot shake the feelings of despair and emptiness. Their negative thoughts about their lives cause them to feel guilty, pathetic and even ungrateful, which in turn causes them to feel worse about themselves and possibly slip deeper into depression.

"There are other people in this world worse off than you." This is another example of a statement that can make a person suffering from depression feel guilty or bad about themselves. Pointing out how well other people deal with their ups and owns only causes your loved one to feel weak and worthless. You may feel as though you are only helping when you say this to your depression loved one, but causing them to feel guilty is not helping. Instead of pointing out other people's strength, try pointing out your loved one's strength. Praise them for what they do accomplish.

"No one ever said life was fair." No, no one ever said life was fair, but that doesn't make dealing with the perceived unfairness any easier. Just knowing that life is unfair will in no way help your loved one to overcome their depression. In fact, thinking about and zoning in on the fact of this unfairness can just cause your loved one to think up more ways in which life is hard, unbearable or not worth living. The mere thought that life is "mean" can spiral them deeper into depression. Instead of pointing out life's unfairness, point out routine things that are good. Do not push your thoughts on your loved one, this can feel like criticizing, but do work positive affirmations into your regular conversation. Point them out as fact and then let the subject drop.

"We all have our crosses to bear." This phrase diminishes your loved one's feelings by insinuating that everyone has something difficult to handle, yet while others are managing to "handle" it just fine, your loved one is not. The message this statement conveys is that you feel as though your loved one should buckle down, face whatever is troubling him or her and then fix it. Depression is not "a cross to bear". It is not a punishment for past sins, or even a fact of life. Depression is a medical illness that can be treated, not an unfortunate incident in life that must be tolerated and dealt with.

Saying anything regarding their depression in anger. Yes, you are going to get frustrated. Yes, you are going to get mad. These feelings are perfectly natural and totally acceptable. What is not acceptable is voicing this anger in a way you won't mean when you calm down, like "I am sick of you and this stupid illness" for example. While it is normal to feel this way, voicing this thought in anger will only push your loved one away and possibly make them feel worse about themselves. When faced with these emotions, stop, take a deep breath and try to rationalize the situation. Force yourself to remember to be angry at the illness and not the person affected by it.

Agreeing with negative views. Fixating on depressing thoughts or worst-case scenarios is often a symptom of depression. While you may feel that you are being understanding by agreeing with them, you could actually be hampering your loved one's progress by perpetuating a cycle of negative thoughts. Next time you are faced with this scenario, try pointing out the realistic view of the situation instead. Do not sugar coat a situation, but also do not allow them to make it out to be worse than it really is. Try to help them put their thoughts in perspective. If that fails, then at least point out the realistic view and then excuse yourself from the conversation. If you continue with a negative thought process, you will only frustrate yourself and enable your loved one to slip deeper into his thoughts.

Changing the subject. It may be tempting to change the subject when your loved one brings up painful thoughts or frustrating emotions, but doing so only causes the sufferer to feel more alone and isolated. Don't be afraid to let them talk about their depression. Talking is a form of therapy and can actually help them to deal with their feelings more productively. You do not have to do anything more than listen for your loved one to reap this benefit.

4

What To Do When Your Loved One Is Depressed.

When a loved one is suffering from depression their moods may change frequently and they may exhibit a lot of despair. They may also suffer physical symptoms that require your help or intervention. During your loved one's harder times, their times of severe, disabling depression, they will need you more than ever before. Although you do not have to become their 24-hour cheerleader, exhausting yourself in your efforts to cheer them up, there are a few key steps that you can take to help them through this trying time.

Be Sensitive. Use your instincts and your personal knowledge of your loved one to read between the lines of his or her behavior. Pay close attention to how what you say and do affects your loved one. Do certain actions or soothing statements work best to drawn him or her out? Does he or she take offense at habitual remarks that come naturally to you? Does your sense of humor, the one your loved one used to laugh at and adore, now make them wince with pain or despair? Watch your interactions with your loved one over the course of a few days or weeks and then use your new found knowledge to determine what works best for you both. Then be sensitive enough to make the appropriate changes for the time being. Also, do not take the need to make these changes personally. Realize that these changes are being brought on by the depression, not a personal grudge against you or your efforts to help.

Be yourself. Sometimes our best intentions do not result in the great outcomes that we imagine that they will. Trying to remain super happy or positive at all times can come off as fake at best, patronizing at worst. Do not feel that just because your loved one is down, that means that you are not allowed to be. Treat your life naturally, experiencing all of its ups and downs. Take care not to focus on or make bigger than necessary the "down" times, but do not pretend that they do not exist either. Your loved one will see through this "my life is perfect, let's concentrate on you" ploy. Your loved one doesn't want a perfect life example. He or she doesn't need to be convinced that your life is perfect in order to believe you can help them. Your loved one just needs you, faults and all. Believe it or not, knowing that you have "bad days" also can help your loved one feel more connected to you and better understood. Be a friend, not a problem solver.

Get them out of the house. Withdraw and self-isolation is a common symptom of depression. A sufferer might try to avoid friends or outside activities in order to hid from their feelings of inadequacy. You can help them by gently encouraging them to get out of the house. By making pleasurable activities available to your loved one, you can help them avoid the trap of "settling into" negative moods or even diminish the chance that these negative moods will take hold of your loved one in the first place. Invite them to dinner or to take a walk or to see a movie. Expect them to resist at first. Be persistent but never forceful. Gradually increasing their social life can give them positive experiences to focus on, and the slow pace in which you do it will give them time to assimilate to new experiences without increasing their stress level.

Get them outside and into the sun. Studies have shown that adequate amounts of sunlight can lighten the moods of people in general, but especially the moods of those suffering from depression. The proven fact that light helps with depression has spurned the introduction of numerous "feel-good" light sources on to the market. While many of these "feel-good light" sources actually do work, the most inexpensive and natural way to get the recommended amount of light is to take advantage of the sun. Not only is it free, easily accessible and readily available, but also spending in time outdoors in the sun also gives you chance to hang out with and connect with your loved. Take simple steps to ensure adequate amounts of sunlight. Move lunch outdoors on nice days, walk to pick your children up from school instead of drive, or ask your loved one to take the dogs for their next walk instead of instantly assuming it will be your responsibility.

Lift their spirits. Everyone, including those suffering from depression, enjoy random acts of kindness. Thoughtful gifts and simple actions can affect your loved one in a big way. Try to come up with small ways to remind them that you love and support them everyday. Write them a letter, give them a back rub, unexpectedly hold their hand, or buy them the latest book or magazine they have been meaning to read. Anything that will bring a smile to their face is always encouraged and no doubt appreciated. Attempt to not make these random acts of kindness seem like a full-blown effort to ease their pain. Make your actions natural; strive to mimic your actions from "pre-depression" times. You want your loved one to feel loved, not pushed to perform.

Be their friend. Spend time with them, talk to them, and show them your support. Many times, when faced with the depression of a friend or relative, people tend to shy away from making contact. They either feel inadequate when they don't know how to help or afraid that they will say or do the wrong thing. The last thing your loved one needs is to feel abandoned. Continue your relationship on the same level it was at before the illness invaded your lives. While you will have moments when you feel anxious or were you feel that you have failed, these moments do not compare to the hurt or shame your loved one could suffer if you chose to give up instead of risk making mistakes. Ease your feelings by understanding that there isn't much you could do to actually harm your loved one if you are trying to be supportive, but giving up on them can, in fact, hamper their recovery.

Let them be. Sometimes the best way to help some one is to let them be. This does not mean that you should abandon your loved one in their times of need, but rather that you should pull away sometimes when you sense that they are getting overly stressed or exhausted. Sometimes the constant demands of trying to "feel better" for other people take their toll and what your loved one needs most is quiet in which to relax in. Alone time is a much-needed luxury for everyone including those that are depressed. Just watch the amount of alone time your loved one receives for signs of social isolation.

Other times, your loved one may feel that it will be nice to have you around enjoying their company but not putting any pressure on them to "explain" or let you "help" with their illness. During these times, resist the urge to discuss the depression or it's effects on your lives.

Stay positive. Even though dealing with the depression of a loved one can be a trying experience, it is best to stay positive when in their presence. This does not mean that you have to stay positive about all aspects of life, just the one's that have to do with your role as caregiver. Your loved one already has enough negative thoughts to deal with. Adding the notion that you are frustrated with them or upset at the situation only leads to further reasons for your loved one to indulge in negative thoughts. People suffering from depression have a tendency to concentrate more on and give more meaning to the negative occurrences in their lives and dismiss or diminish the positive events. Recognize your need to vent about your frustrations or concerns but attempt to save them for times that you are alone or with someone else you can talk freely with.

Do not put too much stock into the negative things that they say when they are feeling down or angry. Many times, when a person is feeling especially bad, they will focus on a topic in which to complain about. This topic can be as serious as the losses they have suffered due to their illness and as simple as the fact that they wanted turkey for lunch and you served chicken. The fact is, if you wait out these minor complaints, the topic will usually pass. Sometimes a depressed person won't even remember being so agitated about the topic in the first place. Other times, one negative topic will be quickly replaced by another one. The point is to not take these topics seriously unless you know for sure that the topics are really important and that your loved one is truly bothered by them. One day you may find your spouse declaring the end of his happiness due to the fact that his favorite book has been lost, only to discover the next day that that book is no longer important and his next crisis is how horrible television programming has become. If you rush out to "fix" every problem that makes your loved one unhappy at any given time, like buying another copy of his favorite book, for example, then you will find yourself failing at every turn and constantly chasing a "simple fix" that can never be found.

Don't let your loved one shop excessively. Trying to elevate one's mood by purchasing numerous products is called a shopper's high. Some people become so addicted to the happy feelings that they get after buying a new item that they begin to buy one item after another in search of a monetary high, never stopping long enough to fully enjoy the last item that they purchased. People who suffer from depression can be more at risk to develop this addiction. If spending money or buying themselves something new temporarily eliminates their bad mood, then they may begin to search out that feeling more and more often. This need to experience a temporary "fix", added to their inability to make sound decisions, can spell disaster. Help your loved one curb their spending habits by taking a tighter reign on their spending cash during times of severe depression. If that is not possible, then you may try accompanying them on their shopping trips to nudge them away from making impulse or expensive purchases.

Believe in them. If you have hope then they can draw hope from you. Just knowing that you believe things will get better, gives them reason to believe they might get better too. Clinical studies show that the odds of recovering from depression are around 80%. With such a large success rate, chances are good that your loved one will eventually feel better. While you do not have to go around proclaiming your belief loudly ever day, just basing your everyday actions on this belief can send a subtle message that your loved one can draw from. Use this knowledge to keep up hope and restore your belief in happy endings, modern science, yourself and each other.

Don't give up. Sometimes a person will need to hear your words of love and encouragement numerous times or even need to hear the words form numerous sources. Even though you may start to feel like a broken record, repeating your words of hope so often that they become habit, don't give up. With persistence and true belief you will eventually happen upon a time when your loved one is well enough to hear the words and actually believe then for themselves. Keep at it!

Make yourself available. Sometimes your loved one might just need someone to talk to or hang out with. Unfortunately these times can be in the middle of the night, while you are at work, or when you are otherwise engaged. Do not feel as though you need to be on call twenty-four hours a day, seven days a week, but do try to make yourself available in their times of need. Luckily, the times that they really "need" you usually won't require much physical exertion. Usually all your loved one will need is a shoulder to cry on or a sympathetic ear. Setting aside time for just the two of you helps cut back on the unexpected needs, but you should expect to be inconvenienced at times. When these times occur, take a deep breath, concentrate on the illness and it's effects on your loved one, and smile or do you best to help them through the crisis without adding any extra pain.

Distract them. When negative thoughts or feelings of worthlessness are weighing on their minds, it may help to have some distraction. Watch their favorite comedy with them, do a crossword puzzle, flip through an old yearbook. The activity itself is not important. The important thing is to choose an activity that will engage them and help draw them out of their negative thought pattern. Do not broach this approach as a distraction though. If you point out your attempts to cheer you loved one up, they may take this as a sign that they are not trying hard enough or feel undue pressure to cheer up since you are trying so hard. Attempt to make these moments of distraction as natural as possible so that your loved one will feel safe and comfortable enough for the distraction to do its job.

Also, do not despair if the distraction doesn't work. Sometimes, the illness itself can make it impossible for your loved one to enjoy anything. Do not push and do not question their feelings. Instead put the activity on the back burner and remind yourself to try again in a few days.

Help your loved one chart their moods. This activity will certainly not put a smile on their face but it is important just the same. By tracking a person's up and downs a pattern can sometimes be determined. Does your loved one suffer more disabling moods in the winter? Are they more irritable around the holidays? Does having a long weekend elevate their spirits?

Once you identify these times, the pattern can be used to pinpoint triggers that worsen or better their condition. This can help you and your loved one by identifying events that he or she needs to avoid during their recovery and events that they can engage in or expose themselves to in order to help them elevate their mood. This information will also help you plan your daily routine around your loved one and their "low" times.

Develop a crisis plan. People diagnosed with depression, and their family members, should have a crisis plan in place. This plan should cover the steps to be taken in case of an emergency or a serious worsening of symptoms. This plan should also include the names and numbers of every current physician and therapist. In times of severe depression, a person may not realize the need for help, or may lack the motivation and concern to seek it. This is where the crisis plan comes into play. In the event that your loved one is too ill to make the decision to seek immediate help, the plan should spell out the doctors, hospitals and treatments that your loved one should be exposed to. If your loved one ever talks of suicide you should seek help immediately. Contact their doctor, call 911, take them to the emergency room or call 1-800-suicide for further instructions.

Along with the above suggestions, you should strive to stay informed about their condition, constantly seek to further your education on depression and attend therapy or support groups with or without your loved one to ensure that they are receiving your continued support.

5

What To Do If Your Loved One Refuses Your Help.

Shame can often be a symptom of depression. A sufferer can become fearful of being judged or seen as weak. This shame can cause some sufferers to decide to "handle" their problem on their own. If all of your gentle persuasions can not change their mind, then you will have to accept their decision (for now) and find others ways to help them cope.

While they might not accept any concrete help, you can still continue to show your support. If they try to push you away either with their silence or by actually walking away, let them, but not before you voice your concern and reiterate that you will be there for them when they decide they want your help.

Also, you may try discussing how you feel as opposed to forcing them to discuss how they feel. Sometimes just hearing that you too, have moments of insecurity, feelings of worthlessness, or feelings of fear can help your loved one begin to trust you enough to open up. Don't try to rush this process, though. This type of support only works gently and at your loved one's own pace. Strive to use these conversations as a way to gain your loved one's trust and ease their feelings of inadequacy.

Although the thought that they are refusing your help can make you angry and cause you to feel like want giving up, you need to be patient and understanding. Sometimes focusing on the behavior, and realizing that it is the illness talking and not your loved one, can help give you the motivation you need to see the waiting through. This knowledge can even make it easier for you to accept the changes that come with your loved one's depression.

Another thing you can do if your loved one won't accept your help is to at least try to persuade them to seek professional help. Sit them down and explain that you respect their feelings and that you will not push them to talk to you about their feelings if they do not want to, but insist that it is crucial that they talk to someone. If they won't agree to professional help, suggest that they talk to a different friend or family member. It may be hard to accept that your loved one doesn't want to confide in you and would rather talk to someone else, but remember…this is not about you or your feelings. This is about helping your loved one to get better. Put your feelings aside for the moment. Once they have recovered, the unselfishness of that act will make your bond even stronger.

If they still won't agree to seek help, research depression and leave the information where they will find it. Sometimes having access to the information and the time alone to process it all will give your loved one the push they need to realize that they are ready to seek help. If nothing else, the information may help your loved one realize that their depression is a medical illness and that realization will give them the confidence they need to overcome feelings of embarrassment or weakness long enough to seek the proper treatment.

If all else fails, find and attend a support group for family members of depressed loved ones. These groups can offer you advice on how to convince your loved one to seek help and suggestions on how to cope when they won't seek it. Plus, these groups are made up of real people facing the same frustrations and feelings as you are. Just talking to someone who understands can help relieve some of the pressure that you are under.

6

The Importance of Family and Friends to Someone Who Is Depressed.

During bouts of depression a person can feel alone, isolated and worthless to the outside world. During these times your loved one needs you more than ever. Just having someone to believe in them and stand by them through their worst times can do wonders to improve a sufferer's feelings of self worth. Along with unconditional love, there are a few other ways that family and friends can be of great importance during a person's road to recovery.

Sometimes a family member or close friend, other than the one responsible for the day-to-day caregiving, is the first to notice that a person is not acting like their usual self. At these times, the caregiver may be too involved to spot slight changes. In that case, an outside friend or family member can play a key role in helping the sufferer and the caregiver to recognize when a medication change may be necessary or when some other aspect of the treatment needs to be changed.

Family and friends can also help by offering to hang out with or talk to your depressed loved one, especially if one of them has suffered from depression themselves.

Throughout depression and the recovery from it, a loved one may encounter escalating medical bills or numerous days off of work. Family and friends can pitch in during this time and ease the financial burden of a loved one diagnosed with depression. Financial assistance can be given to buy medications, pay co-pays for doctor visits, support loved ones during employment lapses and in the form of extras or little indulgences that can serve to lift your loved ones spirits. Financial assistance should never be given in a way that allows a depressed person to give up trying and concede to relying on help, but financial help should be offered and may even be necessary when a loved one is working at recovery but falling on hard times. Since the day to day caregiver will be expected to handle the brunt of these expenses, it will be nice to have other concerned family members or friends that want to help. If numerous people are involved in the financial support of a severely ill loved one, then the financial burden and the worries that accompany it can be lighted for all involved.

7

Taking Care Of Yourself (So You Can Take Care Of Them).

Finding ways to take care of yourself both physically and emotionally is as important to your loved one's well being as it is to yours. If you become ill or depressed yourself, you will no longer be able to take care of your loved one as successfully.

According to the National Institute for Mental Health, caregivers spend about 21 hours taking care of their loved one each week. If a caregiver doesn't work outside the home that number can increase tremendously. Add those hours to the hours a caregiver spends doing "normal" things like shopping, cleaning, sleeping and taking care of other family members and you have the perfect recipe for stress related illness. To raise your energy level and avoid feeling resentful of your role and your depressed loved one, it is imperative that you set aside time to nurture your mind, body and spirit.

The first thing you should do as a caregiver is join a support group. By talking to others that are going through the same thing that you are, you can begin to understand that you are not alone after all. This understanding can go along way toward making you feel nurtured when you are used to doing all the nurturing for someone else.

If meeting once a week at a location away from home is inconvenient, then you should look into joining an online support group. These groups usually have twenty four hour, seven day a week accessibility and come with the added convenience of links to other information and resources.

If talking to strangers makes you nervous or uncomfortable, then you should at least seek out friends that have had a similar experience. Talking and spending time with "regular" friends is important, but conversing with those that truly understand your situation is more helpful when you are trying to sort out your emotions or you are just feeling frustrated and guilty and you need someone to vent to.

In place of a support group, you can also seek therapy for yourself. The constant struggle to help someone through depression can take its toll on your emotions. Having a professional to talk things out with can help you put your feelings into perspective and give you a resource if further treatment is needed.

The following is a list of other actions you can take to keep yourself healthy and happy in your role as caregiver.

Understand and accept your feelings. Remind yourself that any feelings you have, no matter how bad they may seem to you, are natural and acceptable. As some point during your role as caregiver you will feel anger, resentment and feelings of ill will toward your loved one. Do not beat yourself up over these feelings. Admit them, accept them for what they are…legitimate, passing emotions, and then move on. To convince yourself that your feelings are normal, share your feelings with a therapist even if you are afraid. Their perspective and knowledge can help you accept your feelings.

Expect ups and downs. It is the natural cycle of depression to result in good days and bad days. Understand that your feelings will be easier to accept during your loved one's "good" days and forgive yourself for any "bad" thoughts on his or her down days. Just as their emotions fluctuate, so will yours as you navigate and encounter their ever-changing needs and behaviors. No good can come from your feelings of self-doubt. Ease up on your expectations and just do the best you can.

Expect your feelings to change. It is not unheard of for a caregiver's feelings to change as the illness continues or even as the hours go by during a particularly bad period. It is natural to start of with a positive attitude and feelings of hope only to have those emotions crushed and changed as your efforts to help go unheeded. When you find your reserves weakening, attempt to bolster your mood with positive thoughts and reminders that things will get better.

Grieve for your loss. People never stop to consider that living with and caring for a depressed person can bring on feelings of grief, this emotion is usually reserved for those dealing with the loss of a loved one. But it is perfectly nature to grieve for the time and accomplishments that are lost to the depression. Small things like vacations, time spent enjoying life together and achievements at work or in your personal life can be lost or at least put on the back burner during a loved one's depression. It is not only helpful to deal with these losses, but it is recommended. Take some time to grieve, wallow in self-pity, and even scream at the unfairness of it all. Then, wipe your tears, accept your current situation and allow yourself to conceive new dreams and aspirations for the future.

Set limits. Although caring for your depressed loved one can sometimes feel like a full time job, you need to set limits on what you can and will do in order to avoid exhaustion and caregiver resentment. Not only will these limits help you, but they will also help keep your loved one from becoming completely dependent by giving them small responsibilities that allow them to build and maintain their feelings of self-worth. Obviously, your limits will be stretched on extremely bad days, but for good days try to maintain control of your limits. Do not allow yourself to fall in to the "overly helpful" trap. If your loved one is capable of making their own dinner, let them. Do not pick up unnecessary chores just to be nice. Be nice enough to let them prove their strength.

Take "time out". Allowing yourself a few minutes each days or a few hours ever week to refresh your spirit and your mind will allow you to continue the care of your loved one for longer periods of time. Pamper yourself with a good book, or a coffee break with a funny friend.

Time-outs can also be a big help when used at times of high emotion or anger. Taking a few minutes during these periods will allow you and your loved one to calm down and sort through your feelings before speaking out of anger or resentment. You may even find that you were wrong in your thoughts and there will be no need to discuss the incident at all.

Accept help. Throughout the months of treatment and recovery, other friends or loved ones may extend a general offer to help. Do not be afraid to accept help or feel that you shouldn't need help. Everyone needs help and it doesn't make you a failure to accept it. Once you are comfortable with accepting help, don't just agree to accept it, instead, offer concrete suggestions for ways they can help. Ask them if they can pick up groceries for you, or take your loved one to the movies so you can have some time to yourself. Most people want to help but just don't know how to do it. Take the pressure off of them by telling them how they can be of the most help to you and your loved one. You might even go as far as compiling a list of "wants" and letting your friends or family members chose the activities they wouldn't mind taking on.

Do not put your life on hold. Many caregivers fall in to the trap of thinking that they need to extend all of their energies into helping their loved one get better. This is a noble thought but one that will absolutely not work for very long. Although depression takes over you life it does not stop it. In order to keep your spirits high and your body healthy, you need to continue on with your own interests, friends and general life. Keeping up with your own agenda will also help squelch feelings of resentment. Do you have a card game scheduled once a month? Do you and your friends get together once a week for dinner out? Of so, continue these engagements unless an emergency comes up. If not, start a monthly activity and give yourself permission to enjoy it.

Have hope. With the right treatment and medication, depression will get better. Read other people's happy-ending stories, talk to patients that have overcome depression, review information about the recovery from depression. Do anything you can to preserve your hope for a happy, depression free future.

Get enough sleep. Sleep is your body's chance to heal itself from the day-to-day pressures of stress and life in general. Without enough sleep, you body will be unable to fight the effects of stress and repair the damage it has caused. Get at least eight hours of sleep as often as possible and nap during the day throughout times of exhaustion and stress. If sleep evades you, take measures to induce drowsiness. Take a warm bath; play relaxing music, read until your eyes grow heavy. If all else fails, discuss the use of over the counter sleep aids with your family physician. Do not be afraid to take such extreme measures. Sleep is really that important.

Eat right. A nutritious, healthy diet is critical to your health, especially during times of high stress. When your body is stressed or over-worked, it uses more vitamins and minerals to heal itself and survive the prolonged periods of increased adrenaline. Make time for at least three well-rounded meals a day, and force yourself to snack on nutritious foods when you are feeling down or tired. Mid-day slumps are your body's way of telling you that it is lacking certain nutrients.

Also make sure you drink sufficient amounts of water. The body needs water in order for vital organs to operate at maximum efficiency and the body also uses water to flush out any build up of toxins produced by stress. Plus, water can make you feel energized.

Exercise. Exercise will not only help your body stay healthy enough for you to take care of your loved one, it will also help your mind stay healthy too. Exercise increases the release of "feel good" chemicals in the brain, bringing about a feeling of well-being and accomplishment. Exercise also lowers stress hormone levels in the blood and increases energy, two benefits that you will invariable need throughout your loved one's road to recovery.

And physically, exercise increases heart, immune system and joint health, all systems that can suffer ill effects during times of stress.

Relax. Relaxation can be just as important to your health as exercise. Periods of relaxation or meditation can lower the levels of the stress hormone, cortisol, in the body, slow body functions such as breathing and heart rate, increase immune function and clear your mind allowing for better concentration and decision making. Build mini-relaxation times into your daily routine. Read a book; take a bath by candlelight, practice deep breathing exercises. Find something that you enjoy and indulge in it for at least fifteen-minute intervals at least twice a day.

Take vitamins. Stress, mental exhaustion, worry, lack of healing sleep and poor eating habits can rob your body of much needed vitamins and minerals. Prolonged exposure to a deficiency of these key nutritional items can cause disease and illness in the body. Optimally, you would strive to meet your body's daily nutritional requirements with health food and diet. Unfortunately, that is not always possible when caring for a loved one that is suffering from depression. Long days and the need to steal moments of alone time may force you to choose other activities when food is what your body really needs. Help combat this unhealthy pattern by adding a multi-vitamin to your daily ritual. In a health conscience world such as ours, there is no lack of specialty vitamins on the market now days. Scan the aisles or ask your pharmacist or physician for a recommendation. They should lead you to a multi-vitamin whose ingredients are specifically combined for your needs and body.

Rest when you are ill. With time demands being issued from your depressed loved one, your other family members and your job, you may feel as though rest is a luxury not a necessity, but rest becomes extremely important when you are feeling ill. Whether your symptoms are brought on my the common cold or a hint from your body that you are working to hard, you need to heed your body's signals and rest in order to give it time to heal. Lack of recovery time from an illness can lead to more serious symptoms or even hospitalization. So the next time you are sick, but convinced that you do not have the time to stop for your illness, remind yourself that you will have to stop for longer if your symptoms turn serious. Head of this scary situation by taking the time for bed rest the next time you are ill.

Watch for signs of depression in yourself. Many caregivers never give a moments thought to the fact that they, too, could develop depression. Unfortunately, statistics of that happening are high. Exam the facts. Depression can be genetic, it can develop from high stress or environmental triggers, it can develop in small stages that are hard to diagnose or determine. Now exam your situation. Your loved one, who is probably a family member, is depressed. Your life is full of daily stress. You are grieving and suffering negative emotions stemming from your loved one's depression on a daily basis. The conclusion…your life is full of the exact predeterminations theorized to bring about depression.

Knowing this and armed with the information you now have about this illness, you should keep a close look out for the signs in yourself. If you notice any of the signs or just begin to feel "empty" or not your usual self, you should seek an evaluation from your physician to rule out any other causes or illness and begin getting help right away.

Make time for your medical appointments. This advisement goes along with the prior one but takes it a step further. With all of the medical appointments and daily demands associated with caring for your loved one, you may be tempted to let your own health maintenance slide. This is a huge no-no. Simple check-ups, yearly physicals and even dental and eye appointments should be scheduled and kept. Early detection of any condition is always best, so the making of and keeping of appointments, even if you do not feel ill, is of extreme importance.

Journal your thoughts. Sometimes, the act of writing things down, gives your mind permission to let your worries or concerns go. Journalizing your feelings, especially the bad ones, can be a great way to achieve this sense of release. Buy yourself a fancy journal, one that matches your personality, and make it a habit to record your thoughts and actions on a daily basis. Many people find that writing in their journal before bed helps them clear their mind enough to fall asleep, but you can use your journal to help your relax and make sense of your emotions at any time throughout the day when you need a mental break.

Writing down your thoughts can help you to put your emotions in perspective. Many times, a situation will seem worse in your mind than it really is. Writing down your feelings helps you sort through the perceived consequences and see events for what they really are.

Writing in a journal also works to give you hope in that you can read past journal entries along the way and see, in writing, the improvements that you and your loved one have made.

If writing in a journal seems to time consuming or you are just not a dairy type person, then you can get the same results by writing your concerns on slips of paper throughout the day. At the end of the day, review these concerns and emotions, make an effort to see them in a realistic light and then tear them up and throw them away. Sometimes, the act of tearing up your negative thoughts and disposing of them in a physical manner will help you to process those thoughts and rid yourself of them in a mental manner.

Seek out "I deserve it" perks. A great way to prevent frustration and resentment is to acknowledge your hard work and daily effort by allowing yourself little rewards. No matter what your job in life, be it a corporate salesman, a schoolteacher, or a caregiver to a depressed loved one, everyone wants and needs confirmation of a job well done. Unfortunately, in the case of a caregiver, you may be the only one capable of handing out that thanks. So, take pride in your efforts and "thank" yourself with a small reward. These rewards can be anything you want, but the best rewards are those that add to your sense of well-being. Buy yourself a new book, some candles to add to your relaxation baths, an hour massage, or even a gym membership to help with your workouts. Enjoy your rewards and partake of them often, you deserve it.

Keep a sense of humor. The ability to keep a sense of humor, during even the roughest parts of life, can literally save your life. Laughter increases endorphins in the brain, bringing about feelings of relaxation and healing effects on stress related illnesses. When a person's body is relaxed and "good chemicals" are allowed to flow through the blood, the body is better able to repair damage and fight infection and disease.

While finding something to laugh about during times of your loved one's severe depression can be quite impossible, it will be worth the effort. Watch a funny movie, browse the humor cards at your local grocery store, listen to or tell a funny story. Sometimes, the latter suggestion can work best of all. Describing an event that happened to you can sometimes force you to see the humor in the situation, especially if someone else notices the humor first. And, hearing a humorous description of someone else's bad day can lighten your mood and help you see the humor in yours.

8

Who Is The Average Caregiver?

By general definition, the term caregiver can apply to anyone who assists someone who is suffering from an illness or is in some way disabled or incapacitated. Caring for someone who is in the throes of severe depression is a perfect example of this definition.

More specifically though, statistics show that the average caregiver is female, over 35 years in age and working outside the home.

According to recent statistics (gathered by FCA, the Family Caregiver Alliance organization, www.caregiver.org) 52 million family caregivers provide care to persons 20 years old or older who are ill or disabled, and approximately 75% of those caregivers are female.

Other statistics show that 11% of caregivers are providing informal care for their spouses, that the caregiver role can last anywhere from less than a year to over 40 years and that the average caregiver can expect to spend at least 5 years caring for their loved one.

In relation to caregiver burnout or depression, other studies found that an estimated 50% of caregivers are suffering from depression. Of these caregivers, approximately 49% are females suffering depression due the result of caregiving. It is also noted that caregivers are two to three times more likely to use prescription medication for depression, insomnia and anxiety than the rest of the population.

Aside from national averages…informal, or family, caregivers come in all shapes and sizes. Men can become full-time caregivers, especially in the instances of depression in their spouse. Adult daughters are more likely to become caregivers, often taking the brunt of care for an elderly parent, whether the "patient is her own parent or that of her spouse. Other female relatives, whether it is an aunt, sister or grandmother, often find themselves in the role of full-time caregiver when no other options or family members exist. Adult sons sometimes find themselves in the role of caregiver, especially when they are unmarried and the disabled person is their parent or when it is their child that is suffering from an incapacitating illness.

9

Avoiding Caregiver Burnout

Caregiver burnout is the number one cause of stress related illness in caregivers. Caregiver burnout is described as physical, emotional and mental exhaustion. This exhausted state is usually accompanied by a shift of going from being a caring, positive, loving caregiver to becoming a negative, isolated, unconcerned one. Burnout becomes an issue when caregivers do not get or accept enough help with their role or try to do more in their role, physically, emotionally, even financially, than they are able. Burnout can also be brought on by feelings of anxiety, depression and stress and guilt in the caregiver. Guilty feelings, stemming from not wanting to take time for yourself at the (unrealistically perceived) expense of their loved one, can bring about the need to push yourself farther and farther until your body collapses in fatigue.

The signs and symptoms of caregiver burnout closely mimic those of stress and depression. These symptoms include…
Social isolation. This symptom is usually noted by the act of withdrawing from friends and family. Wanting to take time to be along is perfectly natural, especially for an over-extended caregiver, but watch for signs of increasing want for time alone, or self-imposed alone time due to other factors such as sadness.
Loss of interest in previous hobbies or enjoyable activities. Caregivers rarely find the time to engage in past hobbies, but if the chance to spend a few hours wrapped up in your favorite past time doesn't perk your interest any longer, you may be suffering from burnout.
Depressed feelings. These feeling include helpless, hopeless or periods of sadness. Watch for signs that these feelings have gone beyond the normal caregiver ups and down and turned into something more serious.

Weight gain or loss, or changes in appetite. While weight gain or loss can be expected if you are missing meals or eating more junk food due to your new role as caregiver, watch for signs of gain or loss that can not be attributed to changes in your diet.

Loss of sleep, or the need for too much sleep. This can include a change in sleeping habits, early morning waking or the inability to fall asleep at night. While these changes will be normal and explainable most of the time, watch for instances where you are feeling better or more relaxed than usual and still suffering from the above sleep disturbances.

Reoccurring illness. Illnesses such as the common cold, or pains such as headache or digestive problems can occur more often or at greater degrees when a person's immune system is compromised due to stress and exhaustion.

Irritability. Fatigue, stress and feelings of sadness can work together to bring about feelings of irritability or anger in caregiver's who have done too much for too long.

Caregiver burnout most often occurs when a caregiver is so busy caring for others that they ignore their own physical, emotional and spiritual needs. Other feelings, such as role confusion, can also aid in developing burnout. Role confusion becomes a problem when the caregiver can no longer distinguish between their role as caregiver and their role as friend, parent, or spouse. At times of great responsibly for the depressed loved one, caregivers can forget that they are a separate person and begin to feel as though their only "job" is to see after their ill loved one's needs.

Unrealistic exceptions can also lead to the feelings and symptoms associated with caregiver burnout. After putting in numerous hours of care and giving an abundance of positive thoughts to their loved one, many caregivers are distressed to find a less than positive outcome from their efforts. Many caregivers expect to see an immediate improvement in the health and happiness of their depressed loved one and become concerned and frustrated when those improvements don't happen over night.

Caregiver burnout can also be brought on by the feeling of lack of control. Lack of money, resources, outside help and knowledge of the illness can bring about frustration and thoughts of failure.

Sometimes, a caregiver can increase their chances of burnout by placing too many demands on themselves. If a caregiver becomes convinced that they are the "key" to their loved one's recovery, or that it is their exclusive responsibility to help their loved one through their ordeal, they can unintentionally set themselves up for failure and feelings of inadequacy. Also, if too many responsibilities are self-imposed, a caregiver will suffer from exhaustion.

It is imperative that caregivers watch for signs of caregiver burnout. Many caregivers, who are currently suffering from burnout, fail to recognize the signs and eventually reach the point where they are unable to care for their loved ones due to their own illness.

Fortunately, there are several ways to avoid or lessen the chances of developing caregiver burnout.

Make an effort to confide your feelings and frustrations with being a caregiver to a trusted friend or family member. Try to choose a friend that truly understands your situation in order to avoid judgement or misunderstandings that can further your feelings of guilt or resentment with your role. If you don't feel comfortable enough to discuss your situation with friends, or you do not want to put any more of a burden on other family members, then seek out a counselor or therapist to share your feelings with.

Be realistic about what you can do for your loved one. Do not take on more than you can handle. Examine and accept your limits, then use those findings to tailor your care for your loved one in a way that benefits you both. Also, be realistic about the outcome of your help. Understand that it will take time for your loved one to recovery, even if you help him or her tremendously.

Schedule in daily time to break away from caregiving. In order to keep your own life in perspective and to feel important as a whole person, not just a caregiver, you need to take time to do things that remind you that you have your own life. Pursue your own interests, ones that have nothing to do with your loved one or their depression. Take a class, learn a new skill, or do something creative to build up your feelings of self-worth and independence.

Learn everything you can about your loved one's depression and use that information to develop new and better ways to help them, thus saving yourself from putting effort into ineffectual methods and time-consuming plans.

10

Thoughts and Concerns From Caregivers.

In this chapter I have included some thoughts from actual caregivers and a few insights of my own. I have been in the caregiver position with my son for over five years now. Three years ago he was diagnosed with Bipolar II Disorder. While he does have "normal" periods and manic periods along with his depression, I have always found the depressive phases to be the hardest to deal with. There is nothing more heart wrenching than loving someone so completely yet still being unable to make his or her pain go away. In light of my experience, I have taken the liberty of expanding on some of the often-spoken concerns I have heard from other caregivers.

"I am embarrassed about my loved one's depression."—Many times throughout your loved one's depression you will encounter people who do not understand this illness. These people will be quick to offer their thoughts and insights. If their opinions are bad, say they believe that depression is a weakness, then you may be embarrassed to discuss your loved one's condition with them. You may feel as though you have to downplay your loved one's symptoms or dismiss the discussion in order to avoid having that person insult your loved one or hurt your feelings. Or maybe you are embarrassed about your loved one's condition because you, yourself, don't understand it. Feeling this way is understandable, but usually avoidable. To solve your dilemma, educate yourself and others about depression. The more you know, the more you will understand and be able to explain.

"I sometimes feel like packing up my things and running away from it all."—This is a common thought among caregivers, especially frustrated, exhausted ones. The feeling of needing to run away can stem from not giving yourself enough down time or "me" time, or from the feeling that your loved one's condition is never going to end. Schedule some extra relaxation in to your day, or better yet, take a mini-vacation. Go away…to the mall, a restaurant, a spa, anywhere as long as it's away from home. While you are there, clear your mind and imagine yourself on an exotic vacation. This visualization can help increase your feelings of "getting away from it all".

"I want my normal life back."—With all the stress and expectations forced onto a caregiver, there may times when they feel as though they are on a path that never ends. The world of a caregiver is far different than the world in everyone else's reality. Knowing this makes it completely acceptable to have periods where you wish you could have you former life back. Accept these feelings, even go as far as allowing yourself to daydream about having different circumstances, then see them for what they are…a way for your mind to deal with your situation, and then take concrete action to build little "old life" routines into your daily schedule. These familiar routines will offer comfort in times of extreme stress and act as a gentle reminder that life will get better and eventually return to normal.

"I get so angry, and then I feel horrible."—Anger is to be expected and it doesn't make you a bad person. Your feelings of anger probably stem from the fact that you are feeling some resentment about the changes in your life. These feelings can also stem from your loved one's perceived lack of motivation to get better. Acknowledge your feelings, attempt to express them to anyone other than your loved one and then forgive yourself for feeling angry.

"I feel guilty all the time."—Guilty feelings can stem from thoughts that you are not doing a good enough job, not feeling as though you are doing enough for your loved one and from complaining about your situation or your loved one's illness or actions, whether out loud or to yourself, when you feel deep down that your loved one's predicament is obviously worse than your own. Guilt can be a good thing when it stems from actual slights and gives you the push you need to achieve better. But, guilt can be a bad thing when it stems from unrealistic slights and it causes you to feel bad about yourself when you are actually doing your best. Examine your feelings of guilt for realistic slights and then do what you can to improve in areas that are really slacking and accept your efforts in areas of your care that are fine. No one can do everything. Allow yourself to be human.

"Will this ever end?"—The duties associated with being a caregiver often extract a heavy toll on your well being, sometimes causing you to give up hope of better days. The best thing to do in this instance is remember that the chances are great that your loved one will recovery and that things always seem worst when you are right in the middle of them. Read past journal entries if you have them, or discuss your feelings with a friend, to help you realize the improvements that you and your loved one have made so far, and to bring back your belief in a brighter future.

"Why can't people be more understanding?"—Along with your regular duties of caregiving, you may find yourself in the role of advocate as well. Since many people will not understand your loved one's illness, it may be up to you to educate them. This education could be as simple as explaining depression to friends or as complicated as having to provide brochures and other depression information and research to your loved one's school, office or primary care physician. Although the role of advocate consumes a lot of time and effort, the results are worth it if the information can help others to help your loved one.

"I can never plan ahead because I never know what each new day will bring."—With each new day bringing new emotions from your loved one and a new set of "needs" that must be met, many caregivers begin to feel overwhelmed. With every activity that gets planned and then changed, caregivers may find their to-do list getting longer and longer with no sign of an end in sight. While a person's degree of depression may keep them from accomplishing certain things on any given day, for example, attending a family gathering or not being able to pick the kids up from school, it is possible to plan things around your depressed loved one in a way that will ease your burden when your loved one is unable to help with general responsibilities. If you need an errand run or a job completed but are afraid to leave the responsibility with your loved one in fear that you may have to change your plans to get it done, ask another family member or friend to help out instead. You can also make it a habit not to plan anything that will require more time than you have to spare in the event that your loved one is having an extremely bad day. As for not being able to plan your routine due to your loved one's "down" moods, that will not change until their therapy and medication take effect. But have hope; there will come a time when life finally slows down for you both.

"When he gets down about or fixated on something that happened years ago, I just want to give up!"—One of the symptoms of depression is the tendency to fixate on negative thoughts. These thoughts can be new occurrences or memories of events that happened years ago but just happen to come to mind. When this happens, just keep in mind that your loved one's mood will pass or at least, that this particular topic will pass. Try to keep their statements in perspective and be patient. Don't agree with the statements if they are unrealistic, but also don't try to talk them out of their feelings. Be there for them and let them vent or acknowledge their feelings then occupy yourself with something else until the topic is exhausted.

"I sometimes resent my loved one because I feel as though I am doing all the work, chores, and other responsibilities on top of trying to be positive for their sake!"—This is a typical comment from caregivers and a very natural one. It is completely acceptable for you to feel this way because as the caregiver, your responsibilities have increased tremendously and it may seem at times like your loved one is not doing enough with the household responsibilities or even their own treatment. To put your resentments in a more realistic light, review the symptoms of depression and remind yourself that your loved one is not purposely avoiding these responsibilities. During times of severe depression, a person can become physically unable to accomplish certain chores or have an extremely difficult time rallying the motivation necessary to get these things done.

"I worry about our finances"—Many caregivers find that they are spending larger amounts of money since they have taken on the role as caregiver. Financial support often takes place in the areas of money for food, medications and cash support for their depressed loved one. Along with this increase in out going cash comes a decrease in cash flowing in. Many caregivers loss income due to arriving late, leaving early or missing days or weeks from work. Caregivers also sometimes find themselves in the position of having to pass up advancements or decline special projects that could include a raise in pay due to the extra time demands placed on them by their loved ones. This upside down balance in financial safety often causes concern for the caregiver who can wonder what the future holds. To help with this concern it is suggested that caregivers increase their savings plans, discuss and search for aid in the form of social security or other social services and take measures to protect their job, such as applying for FMLA (Family and Medical Leave Act). FMLA is a government mandate that calls for employers to protect their employees' jobs by offering them up to 12 weeks of unpaid time off per calendar year to care for ill or disabled family members.

Being honest about and accepting your feelings, even if you deem them as wrong, can help you to face them, deal with them and then dispose of them. If you can't express your concerns to your friends, at least express them in therapy. Studies have shown that when support groups, therapy and down time are used in conjunction, caregivers are more likely to be less stressed, more satisfied with their role as caregiver and more likely to be able to continue their role as caregiver for a longer period of time.

11

How Your Loved One Feels.

(Thoughts and Advice From Those Who Suffer From Depression)

Reading these thoughts and comments may be hard, especially if your loved one is currently depressed, but they are included here for a very important reason. Just as you need to know that your feelings are normal and that others feel the same as you do, you also need to know how your loved one feels and know that their feelings and emotions are also normal and, more importantly, real. While the following comments may seem dire or scary, it is important to hear how the disease feels from someone who is actually suffering from it. As you read the following comments, don't judge, get scared, or loss hope. Use the statements to explore your loved one's emotions and hopefully build a better understanding of the pain they are experiencing.

With their terrific honesty and candor, the sufferers who chose to share their feelings have made it possible for others to get a glimpse inside a life with depression. (Note: These statements were taken from many discussions in different scenarios. Some of the sufferers shared their opinions in emails, while others shared in person at support groups. Some names have been changed or left as anonymous for privacy reasons).

"When I am depressed everything seems like a chore. Just the thought of having to do something, evening talking to a friend, seems so overwhelming. It gets to where I feel so tired and life just seems to pass by in a blur."—Pat

"Please don't ever tell me to cheer up. Do you think I actually like feeling like this? What's worse is knowing you want me to cheer up and not being able to. I end up feeling like I am letting you down and that just makes me feel worse."—anonymous

"Don't ask me why I am depressed or why I am feeling this way. I DO NOT KNOW! I just feel sad, or more correctly, numb, and I have no idea why."—Jim

"I am scared. Scared that I will never get better. Scared that each new medication or therapy won't work. Scared that I will loose you. Scared that this will be my life. Scared to give up, but scared to hope. I'm just scared."—anonymous

"It's not that I am sad so much, it's more like I feel no desire to do anything…everything about my life and the world in general feels flat, bland."—anonymous

"I am ready to give up. My only options seem to be living with this horrible feeling everyday for the rest of my life, or ending it now. I am tired of fighting this."—anonymous

"One of the phrases that I hear from my friends that sets my teeth on edge is this: "But Roy, you don't SEEM depressed. You're doing SO MUCH! Maybe you're just a bit down?" Aaaaaaaargh!!!!"—Roy

"I feel weak…and embarrassed. It always seems as though others can handle their problems better than I can. Then that makes me feel like a failure, or worse feel as though you think I am a failure."—Tom

"I feel like no matter how hard I try, I can't please you. I know you love me and want me better, but I can't seem to make it go away and I can't tell you how it feels. I see your frustration with me in your eyes."—Sara

"I am tired of people looking at me like I could stop this if I wanted to. Having everyone treat you like a loser takes away your will to try."—anonymous

"I truly want your help, anybody's help. I just don't know what to ask for. I have no idea why I feel this way so how is anyone else going to know?"—anonymous

"I feel betrayed. Betrayed by my mind, by my body, by medical science. Nothing I say, feel or do seems to make this problem go away."—Chris

"I am frustrated. I am used to being able to control my life and my emotions. I get so angry when my brain won't work like I want it to. I feel lost, confused and scared."—Tina

"Just getting out of bed each day takes so much effort and motivation. Motivation I don't have and effort I can't see using just to face another horrible day."—anonymous

"I often get the thought in my head that life would be better for everyone if I just disappeared. The hurt that I am causing everyone makes me feel so guilty."—anonymous

"I would like people to simply hear me, and use reflecting techniques to demonstrate to me that they've heard me. (I had a girlfriend who was depressed, and this tool worked for her too. And it's also worked with bipolar friends of mine when they've been in a down cycle.) Reflecting is very easy, but for some reason, people feel very self-conscious about doing it, and they assume that they're not being helpful.

Here's what I mean by reflecting. Look interested in hearing what I'm saying. Make non-vocal signals to show that you're hearing me. For instance, the odd nodding of a head, eye contact, positive body language, a few "aha", "yeah?" "oh", "hmmmm" go a long way. Every now and again, for you to say, "Can I just summarize what I'm hearing? You're saying, that you feel trapped, unlovable, as though you have no energy. Is this right?" Then SHUT UP and allow me to continue. If I'm crying, please don't try and make me laugh or smile. I'm not crying as some kind of attempt to test your comic skills. I'm crying because I'm in severe pain. Rather ask if it's okay to hold me, and do so, paying particular attention to whether or not I'm displaying signs of claustrophobia. DO NOT GIVE ME ANY ADVICE. You do not know what this illness is. And even if you're depressed or depressive yourself, there is NO way you're going to prove to me in this moment that you know what I'm going through. Your advice instantly identifies you as someone who wants me to snap out of this. Just don't do it. If you have to say something, say something like this: "I'm hearing that you're depressed. I can't know what that's like for you, but it sounds hard. I'm not going to try and make it go away. I just want you to know that I'm here, judgement-free. I'm your friend, and I love you no matter how you're feeling."—ROY

"I wish people understood that if I seem to be avoiding them or putting them off, it really has nothing to do with them personally, but is a manifestation of the disease. I need a lot of rest and down time. I've learned that I do better if I set limits on myself, avoid tiring myself out, and try to avoid over-committing myself, as that leads to overwhelm. (Still working on this one!)"—Diane

"During my worst days I feel like absolutely nothing is worthwhile. I can find no reason for my continued existence and constantly rehash all the mistakes I've made during my lifetime. It's like wearing very dark sunglasses in a dimly lit room with no windows or doorways. There is no way out. Nothing is clear, nothing is in focus. I know that I need to remove the sunglasses, but it just takes too much effort to even think of trying. Some days it feels like it's too much effort to even breathe and even marveled at how easy it would be to just not make the effort at all."—Jill

"I feel like hell. At worst, I am very aggressive, I think all people, places and things are crap and should be stamped on. I feel claustrophobic, I am bored, I feel helpless, I feel tired but at the same time I am restless so although I feel tired, I am not relaxed enough to lie down and have a nap. I also go into a kind of stupor where I sit there staring into space. I also feel like someone has their hands around my throat, throttling me. I also look at things very negatively and pick faults with everyone and everything."
—Mark

"I wish that people would get this stupid idea out of their head that I can just "snap out of it". I wish they would stop thinking that if I watched some comedy or laughed at a joke that the depression would suddenly disappear. When someone finds out I have depression, their first response is "what are you sad about?" It isn't a case of being happy and sad. It's a case of the body going through severe mood swings and having a giggle or eating a Big Mac isn't going to make me feel any better. To interact with me better, they should understand that I have no control over the depression—when it arrives, it stays until it decides to leave. I can't order it to go. When it comes, the person shouldn't think it's their fault. It isn't! They should also understand that if I can't work, if I can't stop falling asleep or if I can't stop crying then so be it. Leave me to get it all out of my system. Bitching about it isn't going to make me any better any quicker."—Mark

"I think the worse feeling with depression is feeling NOTHING. At least sometimes when I am sad or irritable I feel something, anything. It is the lack of feeling or caring that is the worse of all."—Jennifer

"No, I can't just "cheer up." A "swift kick in the pants" is not what I need. You wouldn't tell someone with arthritis or asthma to "just get over it." Please don't tell me to count my blessings-when I'm able to I will, but when I'm in a depressive episode I can't recognize them. If I want to talk to a shrink, I'll pay someone. You can tell me what works for you, but don't assume it will work for me. You don't have to tiptoe around the issue. All of these are things I would have like to have said to various people at various times. Usually, I don't, though. These remarks would sound surly said out loud, but I do get cranky at a lot of the misconceptions and platitudes."—Sue

"I wish people would understand that when I get grumpy and down, it's not their fault. They don't need to "cheer me up" and they don't need to berate me for not "snapping out of it". I am what I am and if you'll just give me a bit of slack, I can work on getting "back to normal"."—Cheryl

"I feel like I'm at the bottom of the well, shut away in darkness and isolation, but able to see the top of the well and hear the cheerful conversation of "normal" people as they enjoy the sunlight and open spaces. I wouldn't "hurt my feelings any if I got hit by a bus". There isn't, after all, any real need to have me here on this earth, is there?"—Cheryl

12

The Interview

The following interview was comprised from many individual interviews with sufferers of depression or caregivers. The interview also contains a unique perspective from one interviewee, in particular. Bonnie Ursprung is both a sufferer of depression and the caregiver for a daughter (age 15) who also suffers from depression. Ms. Ursprung was diagnosis with depression at the age of 25 and her daughter was diagnosed 6 years ago. Ms. Ursprung currently takes medication for her illness but is not in therapy at this time. The other interviewees chose to change their names or remain anonymous.

This interview was completed and included in hopes of giving the readers a inside view on what living with and dealing with depression can sometimes entail and maybe offer a few tips or realizations from someone in the trenches with the disease.

Jody Ehrhardt: What do you wish people around you understood about your depression and your feelings? For example, if you could tell them a few things that would help them interact with you better, what would they be?

Bonnie Ursprung: I wish that more people could understand that, for some of us, it is not a "mind over matter" issue; We cannot just "think" ourselves happy. Many people assume that medication is never necessary for depression as there are ways to get through what is causing the depression. Unless they have suffered the types we on medications have they have no idea.

If more people could understand that, for the most part, we are normal people it would help. Understand that, sometimes, due to medications (or lack thereof) our moods can swing quite hellishly. Don't let that deter you from getting to know us…our mood swings can be survived. I promise.

JE: Do you feel that the fact that you to also suffer from depression helps or hurts your ability to help your other relatives deal with their illness?

BU: I believe that it helps her, as I can understand that sometimes you are not ready to talk about what has happened to you as it will take you deeper into the recesses of your dark memory. I also understand when feelings simply take over and you cry for no apparent reason. I do not demand a reason why if she says she doesn't know.

JS: Helps. I am the first one facing it out loud which is helping others to realize that they could seek help too and that they can feel better.

JE: What is the most important advice you can give someone who is caring for a loved one with depression?

JS: Don't judge. Encourage the person to have an open conversation about what they are feeling and what they need to do for themselves to get help. Look up information on the disease…talk and confront and take the person to the doctor. It is scary to get out of bed, even scarier to fix what is wrong without support.

S: Ask what the person needs instead of assuming you know. For a while my husband would try to "fix" me or tell me jokes to "cheer me up." Later he figured out that if I was withdrawing, to say, "Is there anything you need?" and "Let me know if there's anything I can do." Quite often the answer is "Give me a hug and then I need to be by myself for a while." Sometimes I can ask for help: "I need to talk about what happened yesterday" or ask him to take on a chore that will relieve some stress.

Once he was able to lure me out of a funk by putting in a videotape of the Mikado, knowing that I can seldom resist it, a comfort film, like comfort food. But that was at the beginning of a downhill slide, not the middle of a full-blown episode. When that happens, I can't even enjoy things I like.

JE: What is the most important piece of advice you have given to your daughter (or another relative) to help her deal with depression?

BU: That everything that has happened to her in her life has made her who and what she is. Everything she has gone through has only made her stronger and that it will all be ok. I have promised her that she will get through this in time and, when she is ready to talk about what happened, I will find her someone if she needs me to. I also suggested that she write in a journal or diary; she has now started writing stories to help cope with a few things (mainly growing up).

S: It wasn't a relative, but I told a friend that she didn't have to have that full-color 3-D and sound video recorder in her head that replayed every stupid thing she ever said or did at random moments, usually the worst possible ones. Then when she got on Prozac I was able to say, "See? I told you that wasn't normal. I knew it would go away." She had to admit that life was better without it. She just hadn't realized that only depressed people have that particular function (or at any rate to such an extreme degree).

I have also told people that when you feel really abnormal, sometimes the best thing to do is something completely normal, like make a cup of tea. It's familiar, routine, and comforting; does not require much energy; and can have a centering effect.

BU: Be patient. You have no better idea than they do what is going on in their head. Dark images and ghosts from the past can easily control them for a short while. If possible get them some form of treatment whether it be medication or therapy if not both to start with. But, over all, be patient.

JE: What frustrates you the most in caring for someone who suffers from depression?

BU: For me it is the fact that, when in the throes of depression, they see no other way than their mind perceives things. They cannot see how things will get better or how lucky they are. Nothing will help them other than letting them cry themselves to sleep on your shoulder. My daughter usually feels better after a good hard cry and a nap.

D: Lack of response. Lack of affect. Lack of visible emotion. When my husband is bothered by depression, he's silent, doesn't feel like doing anything, is unresponsive. I understand completely, but the house often feels like all the air has been sucked out of it. There is so much inertia in a house where two people suffer from depression.

J: Knowing that nothing I can say or do will truly make a difference in how they feel right this minute.

JE: What is something that someone has done for you while you were "down" that really worked to help you or that made the biggest impression on you and your road to recovery?

BU: My ex-husband used to let me cry on his shoulder and he would hold me until I was through it. I have "bad days" and the only thing that helps is the crying although you don't know why. Just support those who need to cry and let them work through it. Hold them and comfort them; it will pass.

J: Oddly enough, it was someone who had absolutely no concept of what depression meant or felt like. He said, "Can't you just snap out of it?" I said something sarcastic like, "Sure, I'll just do that." He went on to research about depression and really tried to understand what it was all about. Just the fact that he made that visible effort and was willing to talk with me about what he was reading, helped. Perhaps because it was tangible proof that someone really did care.

JS: Confronted me. I can be a bear and I am really good at hiding that I am hurt and need help, I think I am ashamed of being weak and I SHOULD be better…but I know it is out of my control and that others do not understand for REAL what I am feeling…almost like I am making a big fat excuse for being depressed and I should be able to do something about it. I need in my life strong people to help me CHALLENGE this feeling. To tell me to shape up by getting help and that it is beyond me…confrontation has been the key to my wellness. Or I should say, the beginning of my wellness.

S: Sometimes it's something really small. Once we were cleaning out the garage and I was starting to dwell on all the reminders of bad years, turmoil, and pain. I remarked that so much of my life had been wasted being depressed and that I regretted all the opportunities I had lost as well as the trauma and distress. My husband said, "But if you hadn't gone through that, you couldn't be as good a friend as you are to H. or R., who are going through it now." It was just the right thing and way different from an abstract "There's a reason for everything."

JE: Can you describe how you feel on your worst days?

BU: My worst days are pretty bad. For most people a bad day simply means having the "blues". Take your "blues" and make them 100X deeper. On a bad day I feel that as if everything is against me: the weather, my co-workers, my boss, my kids, fate, etc. There is the feeling that all anybody wants is to hurt me or is out to undermine my efforts to live a decent life. Then the rage begins to build and I am mad at the world. Anything and everything is subject to my anger and hatefulness. Then comes the, "I'm not worth anything" phase. My kids, my boss, my mother, family and boyfriend all deserve so much better than me. I don't deserve to breathe. I'm a waste of good oxygen. You get the idea.

Sometimes I only go through one or two of those phases before a good hard screaming cry is needed or just happens. Fortunately, my medications keep me out of that frame of mind…. um…when I don't forget to take them. :oops:

JE: How long have you been in therapy for your depression?

BU: Actually I stopped going to therapy for my depression. The day I walked into the psychologist's office and he asked, "So, what do you want to talk about today?" I decided that I could do a better job on my own. My deepest fears and darkest thoughts are buried inside and will not come out on their own. They will have to be dug up and, honest truth, it will not be an easy task.

J: I tried therapy off and on from age 18, but didn't find it to be helpful. I had a "nervous breakdown" on September 19, 1998 and was hospitalized for three days. The staff kept me under suicide watch for 24 hours. My depression deteriorated into a bipolar condition with extreme mood swings. A condition of my release was to attend therapy. The recommended therapy was group sessions, but I proved to be too empathetic with the other patients and my doctor took me out of the program. A suitable therapist couldn't be found in my area, so I was allowed to be on monitored medications. Several years later I did find a therapist, but discovered that talking about the depression actually made it worse. I'm better off dealing with it in my own way.

M: I did one year of therapy last year because the health insurance company demanded it. It didn't work and I ended up having a huge fight with the therapist. He was quick to blame my parents for my problems and I hated that. I don't do therapy now, despite the best attempts of the health insurance company to force me into hospital.

JS: I went on and off every since I was 26. Of course it took a while to find someone worth talking to. I found one therapist that I had for about 5 months. And another I had for about 3 months that were very helpful.

S: I don't remember, it was years. But now I just go to my family physician for medication, dosage monitoring, and the like. I guess I'm in what you'd call the "maintenance" phase.

JE: Do you work outside the home, and if so, what kind of reactions did you receive from co-workers concerning your depression?

BU: Actually, because my mood can change from day to day and hour to hour most of them do not know what to think of me. Only a few people have ventured near long enough to try to figure me out. This, believe it or not, can be a good thing.

S: I've been cautious about whom I reveal it to at work. Most of the time when I do, another person pipes up, "Oh, really? Me too! I've taken Prozac (or St. John's Wort or whatever) for years!" I usually inform my direct supervisor just in case, for example, that if I have to switch medications I may have a few really bad weeks. Mostly I tell them that if I lose my sense of humor or seem withdrawn or antisocial, it will pass in a day or two. (Of course, this is only true since I've been treated and stabilized.) What I don't need is someone trying to take my emotional temperature every day, constantly asking if I'm OK.

JE: Did your husband suffer any consequences at work due to your condition, for example lost hours or passed up promotions?

BU: No. Fortunately he did not suffer any consequences at work because of me. *JE: Where friends, on average, supportive of your condition? Did you lose any friends during this time, or where any relationships weakened?*

BU: Actually my friends were very supportive and understanding. I did not, nor do not, have many who have reached "friends" status as I know the difference between friends and acquaintances. The only relationship that weakened due to my depression was the one with myself before I got on medications. Now I have a strong relationship with myself and know who I am.

J: I've never had any close friends. I think the depression makes me too self-isolated. The one person who tried for a time to be friends and get me out of the house now and again, finally gave up and stopped calling.

JS: My friends have been an amazing source of support. Once I started slowly letting all of them in to know what has REALLY been going on…I have been blessed. Part of my depression is severe irritability and I can be a beast, I am lucky to have people in my life who love me despite of myself! Of course, I have this tendency when NOT suffering from depression…it just amplifies my normal mood when it is clinical.

S: I'd have to say that mostly, they've been great. Of course, a lot of my friends have the same sorts of problems; perhaps we attract each other. I will say that I have noticed that I sometimes avoid one depressed friend when all she can talk about is gloom and misery, and I imagine that other people have felt/done the same about me at times. She resists getting any further help or treatment and it frustrates me. And she may avoid me when I keep suggesting that she get some help or see a doctor about her dosage. But we're part of each other's support system and I can't picture us giving up on one another.

JE: Did you ever feel like "giving up"? And if so, what helped you find the strength to go on?

BU: On the occasions where I do forget to take my medications I do suffer from wanting to give up. The last time it got severe was about 3 years ago and I began making out my Last Will and Testament. Rarely does it get that bad…usually only to the point of my wanting to give up until I look at my girls. That helps a little.

J: I've considered suicide many times, but haven't seriously tried it or I wouldn't be here now. What kept me going was initially my daughter and later, my pets.

M: Now I didn't ever contemplate giving up but at the beginning, yes, I wanted to. I considered suicide twice. What made me go on? I'm not sure. Part of me wanted to beat the depression and not let it win. Perhaps that is stubborn pride. Part of me treasures my life and I reminded myself there was so much more I could do in life if I live. Another part thought of my friends and family being hurt if I did something to myself and that thought alone made me stop any suicidal thoughts.

JS: Nope. Never ever give up. I am not sure where this has come from, somewhere deep inside…the worse I have ever been I thought of not existing and no one would care or notice…but I never ever gave up. I somehow snap out of that deep mood, at least for a little while. I just have some kind of inherent strength that I will get better, someday in the future…and knowing that I made it this far means I will somehow overcome this phase too.

JE: Do you use medication to help your depression? If not, how come? And have you used medication in the past?

J: I have tried numerous medications over the years. Some helped, some did not. I'm not using any medication at the present time and haven't for over two years. I've lived with my depression long enough to know when I can deal with it on my own and when I need help from medication. So far, so good.

JS: Ugh. I have tried and not been compliant. And tried again and not been complaint. And now, for the last month. I am really working on getting better. I hate hate hate the idea that I need a pill to make myself snap out of this…HATE not being in control of my own mind. And I am educated and I know that it is beyond myself and I could help anyone else in the entire world face the facts about depression, but when it has come to myself, I don't believe one single word. I SHOULD be strong, I am making excuses…I don't need medications…this is the hardestpart for me to accept.

S: Absolutely. "Better living through chemistry" is my motto. I've tried about every kind there is and am now settled into a mixture of Lexapro, Effexor, and Buspar, with the occasional Ativan as needed. I am delighted they exist and will happily stay on them the rest of my life. I have no problem with the fact that I need them. Would diabetics resent the fact that insulin keeps them alive?

When I first started on Prozac, though, my mother said, "I've heard that Prozac is a ticking time bomb." "Uh-oh, she's been listening to Phil

Donahue," I thought. "Should I tell my husband to lock up the guns?" I asked her. "Only if he thinks it's necessary," she replied.

JE: How important do you feel diet and exercise is to beating depression?

J: I have no feelings about diet, but exercise is definitely beneficial even if it's simply walking.

JE: How do you stop or decrease negative thinking?

J: For every negative thought I have about myself, I have to think of one positive thing about myself. Sometimes it works, sometimes it doesn't.

C: I was unable to do so when I was severely depressed. When negative thoughts come up now I tell myself it DOESN'T MATTER—concentrate on today and the good things I have: a loving partner, a nice home, a garden to potter in, a cat who sits on my lap and purrs, a friendly neighborhood where people greet each other in the street, just being alive to appreciate all these things.

S: I read a lot, which forces me to concentrate on whatever I'm reading about.

JE: Does anxiety come with your depression?

J: The "nervous breakdown" was preceded by several years of anxiety attacks. I've not had a serious anxiety attack now in several years, thank God. When I'm severely depressed, I'm usually too tired to be anxious about anything…it takes too much effort to care that much about anything.

S: You bet. All the time. Hence the Buspar and Ativan. I can't tell you how or why they're related, though.

JE: Do you belong to a support group? If so, is it in person or online?

JS: This is the odd part. BOTH of the therapists I trusted recommended group therapy for me. And I have resisted greatly. Why? Because I am the person who gets satisfaction with helping everyone but myself. I help others like other people breathe. It is who I am. And in a group?

I would have to admit I am weak and allow others to help me. Not what I am ready to accept. HOWEVER, the interesting twist is I have created my own little support group unknowingly online through my blog. I found that admitting my depression has allowed others to email me and share their feelings. Knowing others DO GET ME and I can still help them by sharing what I have been going through is one amazing process towards my getting better…really, I guess I had to do this on my own though. I am the one in control when it comes to whom I am talking to. (Which might be counterproductive and I should be in group anyhow) but I will face that road when I get to it.

S: No formal group; I don't do well in group settings. I do have an informal group, a circle of friends, support system, call them what you will, but no meetings or anything like that. I tried attending a group, I won't say which one, because it may help others, but found it very weird and definitely not for me.

13

Resources

Many resources exist that can help you and your loved one deal with his or her depression. The trick is knowing where to look. The following is a list of resources and a brief description explaining what kind of help they offer and where to find them.

The phone book: There are many different headings in the phone book that can be utilized to find the help you need. Some popular headings to start with include…"mental health", "social services", "hospitals", "physicians" and "therapist". Mental health and social services listings will give you the names of social workers, support groups, mental health centers and facility run programs. The listings for hospitals, physicians and therapists will give you names and numbers for healthcare professionals in your area.

Your place of employment: Your company or the company of your loved one may have an employee assistance program in place. If so, you would be wise to utilize this resource. This program was started with the intent to help employees through times of crisis free of charge. Sometimes this is just through a telephone consultation and other times the company has a therapist that sees the employees in person. Sometimes this service also offers referrals, educational material and advice on taking personal paid leave.

The Internet: Using a search engine and typing in the word depression can instantly put you in touch with an abundance of resources on the world wide web. These resources range from simple sites that explain depression to more elaborate sites that run message boards, support chat rooms and offer books on the subject of depression. Although most of then are very valuable and easy to use, a few are so helpful that they merit mentioning here.

www.depression.com This site is funded and developed by GlaxoSmith-Kline and hosts a wealth of information pertaining to depression. Tabs located on the home page cover topics such as understanding depression, treating depression and living with depression.

www.nimh.nih.gov/publicat/depression.cfm This site is sponsored by the National Institute of Mental Health. On this site you will find information pertaining to depression such as types of depression, treatments for depression and psychotherapy descriptions. This site also offers information on clinical trials, publications pertaining to depression and information on current research in the field of depression and mental health.

www.psychologyinfo.com/depression/ This site provides general information about depression (its causes, treatments and types) along with information about medications and therapies. There is also a section dedicated to frequently asked questions about depression and a section providing a national directory of psychologists.

www.rxlist.com This site is dedicated to the consumer's research of medications. Consumers can run searches by keyword, drug name, condition, side effect and drug interaction. Each search renders a complete list of information including a drug's brand name, generic name, it's patient information, it's side effects and interactions, it's drug class, it's proper use, storage and more. There is even a link that will return a price quote for certain medications.

www.support4hope.com This site acts as an online support group for sufferers of depression and other mental illnesses. Their format includes a 24-hour chat room, specially scheduled conference chats, a newsletter, forums for discussion and general information about depression and numerous other conditions.

www.depressionfallout.com This site boasts itself as a site completely dedicated to helping...*spouses, lovers, parents, children and friends of those who suffer from depression or bipolar disorder.* The site offers many resources including messages boards, help topics, recommended books and includes a comprehensive list of Internet resources pertaining to depressive illness, those who suffer from them and those who care about the sufferers.

14

Beyond Depression

Right now, your every decision and action is probably bases on what is best for your loved. But, believe it or not, there will come a time when all of this is behind you. For now, use the suggestions covered in this book, seek information and education at every turn and take care of yourself until the depression is in remission.

In planning for your life after remission, remember that recovering from depression will involve many small steps over a long span of time. You may not even notice these changes until your loved one is completely better, that is why it is important to weave "life after depression" routines into your daily life now.

One of the hardest things about your loved one's recovery is re-learning how to live your life. After years of rewriting your life script to include depression and caregiving, you are suddenly free to rewrite it again, only this time you can chose what to include. This prospect can make people extremely happy and scared at the same time. Be patient with yourself. It will take time to learn your new role. And this time it will be your turn to ask your loved one for support and understanding. If you over-scrutinize them when they are sad, jump to conclusions when they are irritable, or assume the worst when they have a bad day…they are just going to have to understand. Seeing as that same behavior has occupied your life for an extended amount of time, it is understandable that it would be too hard to just turn off your emotions like a switch. Accept the great changes in your loved one, the slow changes in yourself and hang in there. After all you have been through the worst and now this is the fun part.

Since you want your loved one's new found recovery to be a time of joy, you will need some tips to help your own "recovery".

Plan and participate in activities that you used to enjoy together. This can be a night of dancing, a big family picnic or even an evening of rented movies and cuddling. Whatever the event, pick it from your past and enjoy!

Take that vacation you planned before your loved one became ill. Now is the perfect time to plan something big and enjoyable. Make it a weekend trip or an all out vacation, just be sure to plan it around a destination you had planned to visit before depression invaded on your lives.

Re-instate that weekly family game night or other ritual you let slide during your loved one's depression. Going back to and actually enjoying old routines can speed up the process of "getting your old life back".

Slowly integrate your old routines in to your daily life, but leave room for new, exciting ones, too. Did your husband used to start the coffee while you retrieved the paper? If so, make that his "job" again. Bringing back old habits can make you more comfortable in your new "old" life.

Take the time to count your blessing. This is probably a habit you knew quite well in your old life, but in your caregiver life you were probably too overwhelmed to do it. Well, now is the time to start again, and this time you will have even more to be thankful for!

Take your time getting used to your new life, enjoy everything, even the "off" days, and most importantly—give yourself a pat on the back. You deserve it! Just look at what you have accomplished. Be proud.

About the Author

Jody M. Ehrhardt is a freelance writer who resides in the Midwest. Prior to starting a career in freelance writing, Ms. Ehrhardt spent nine years in the field of pharmaceutical research. Ms. Ehrhardt currently works for two online magazines, one newspaper in New York and is also the assistant editor and staff writer for her local newspaper. Her book credits include a nonfiction book about Childhood Onset Bipolar Disorder. Ms. Ehrhardt is the mother of a bipolar child and her book, *On the Outside Looking In* is a touching depiction of her family's daily battle with bipolar disorder and the effects the illness had on her entire family. Her approach with the book was to enlighten her readers with the personal, daily battles, both emotional and physical, associated with this disorder, not to just expand on the medical jargon already widely available about this disease.

0-595-34404-6